Taming the Dragon's Tail

Taming the Dragon's Tail:

Growing Ginseng and Goldenseal for Profit

By
Ron von Knasick &
Ann Lee Wynn von Knasick

Aventine Press

Published by Aventine Press
1023 4th Ave #204
San Diego CA, 92101
www.aventinepress.com

ISBN: 1-59330-364-5

Table Of Contents

Introduction

Ginseng is a perennial plant unique among its herb counterparts in its history, medicinal potential, and marketability. The market price reflects the growing demand for this herb as it has increasingly permeated into mainstream American culture in a plethora of products including traditional supplements, cosmetics, ice tea, beer, and even candy. It is however not a new phenomenon, the Chinese have revered it for at least several millennia and it has been traded in North America since before the birth of the United States itself.

Due to this demand there exists great profit potential for those buying and selling ginseng. The crops sold from Canada and the Untied States exceed $25 million annually in value. The only way to sell it is to duly harvest roots growing wild or cultivate it. Culling wild specimens is becoming difficult with wild populations being ravenously decimated in North America and Asia. Therefore this field guide gives the reader the knowledge needed to independently plant, grow, and harvest ginseng.

Furthermore aside from ginseng there is a chapter on growing and selling goldenseal. Goldenseal is currently more valuable than field cultivated ginseng and easier to grow, which makes it an excellent cash crop for diversification of your investment. Growing herbs for profit can be arduous work but also very rewarding, with this guide you will be armed with the tools of knowledge needed to succeed.

Chapter I

Ginseng the Plant

A) History

The name of the Ginseng plant was derived from the shape the root can develop into during healthy growth, this while growing in its native environment (*see* Ginseng Diagram). Smaller roots branching out from the central root could possess the likeness of appendages thus believed by ancient Chinese to resemble the human body and hold healing powers. This reliance, belief, and acceptance of a plant by its looks holding some special power (i.e. possessing a sign from "God"), in Anthropology is known as the Doctrine of Signatures. This concept was active in ancient China, Renaissance Europe, and many other cultures largely until the late 1800s. From this theory and root characteristics, *renshen* (or Man-root) is what the Chinese would come to call it. Phonetically the name then evolved from *renshen* to become *ginseng*.

Anthropological research supports the theory that humans evolved from a primitive hunter-gatherer social structure thus roots were commonly dug and ingested with the diet of the time. It is reputed that against this backdrop the Chinese at an early date were able to deduce the effects of this peculiar looking root and due to its curious shape, early herbalists believed it was of great value to the human body. Historians offer differing dates as to when the Chinese first began using ginseng with appreciable organization but it likely started approximately 3,000 to 5,000 years ago. About 2,000 years ago the use of ginseng was recorded in the Chinese medical treatise *Shen-nung pen-ts'ao-ching* where amongst other claims it stated that protracted use of ginseng would result in a long life. Ironically these claims of longevity, helped increase the value of ginseng resulting in the violent loss of life protecting its growing grounds in conflicts between the Chinese and the Tartars. In an era when illegal possession and trafficking of the root was a capital offense, there is little doubt this root was highly treasured.

Thus the Chinese have ascribed great value to the root ever since early history. To think this root was greatly valued prior to, and while, the Roman Empire was nearing its apex, long before humans invented the plane, split the atom, or sent people into space and onto the moon, is indeed staggering and yet its demand has only grown. Not surprisingly with such a long history of this demand its wild counterparts have nearly been hunted to extinction especially in its natural habitat of China (mainly Manchuria) and Korea. The price paid for existing wild Chinese ginseng presently can be as much as $150 - $450 per gram.

Meanwhile almost 300 years ago, likely traced to the separation of the continents over 149 million years prior, in North America a cousin of Asian *panax ginseng* dwelled and waited to be found. It was discovered to be growing in congruent natural woodland habitats and between the 30 - 50 degree north latitude zones like its Asian counterpart. It became known as *panax quinquefolium* or its common name, North American ginseng. This root was used by some of the native tribes for its presumed healing power, most notably the Iroquois Nation. The "western" discovery and export of North American ginseng can be traced back to two French missionaries.

Ginseng Plant & Root

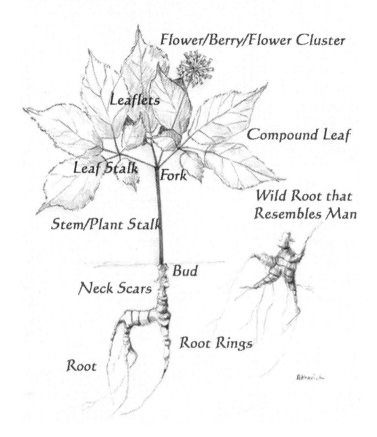

In 1709, Father Jartoux was introduced to Asian ginseng while surveying and traveling through China. Correspondence describing the qualities and characteristics of this revered root had been reported back to Europe. Several years later while working from this body of information, Father LaFitau discovered North American ginseng in Montreal, Canada. Samples were collected and sent to France to be analyzed. By 1718 the Chinese considered the North American species legitimate and trade soon developed. This continued until the wild crops and trade were devastated by over-harvesting, exploitation of premature roots, and carelessness in drying. This engendered a reduction in ginseng harvested from Canada for decades until the practice became popular south of Canada in what was then the British Colonies at which point trade with Asia was rehabilitated. Of course years later the Colonies had their own problems and eventually desired to jettison the tyrannical yoke of Great Britain, which destabilized trade in general and resulted in a revolution.

After the American Revolution (1775 - 1783) trade was again rehabilitated and it is reputed that Daniel Boone in the late 1780s employed Native Americans to harvest the plant in the wild. Ginseng remained a valuable commodity even during the War Between the States (1861 - 1865) in fact exports in the year of 1862 surpassed 300 tons of roots. With increased demand and an appreciable price paid, ginseng was once again nearly hunted to extinction in the westward-expanding American territory that comprised the country in the 1860s just as wild crops were exhausted in the territory that embodied the country during the 1820s.

With wild ginseng being over-harvested and in many cases completely destroyed, the problem arose of how to satiate demand with a disappearing plant population. By the 1890s a man who is worthy of mention and credited for pioneering effective large-scale cultivation of North American ginseng would solve this query. He was a resident of central New York, named George Stanton. He began extracting wild ginseng and replanting it in a controlled environment while adroitly copying the natural environs from which it was removed. From this humble beginning he eventually had over 150 acres of ginseng cultivated and the business blossomed from there.

Today, nearly 300 hundred years since European settlers began harvesting ginseng in North America it is still highly valued and remains threatened in the wild. Ginseng is a protected plant under the Convention on International Trade in Endangered Species. Therefore commercial cultivation pioneered by Stanton is especially important to meet expanding demand and preserve the threatened natural specimens. In the United States, Wisconsin leads the country in commercial ginseng production surpassing every other state where it is cultivated. While presently Kentucky remains the largest producer of harvested wild roots that are properly documented.

Today gardens have sprung up in virtually every region of the United States even Arizona and northern Florida. The export of commercial ginseng creates a buoyant market that has been growing yearly and is estimated to soon exceed $25 million from North America.

As an interesting note, when westerners became more familiar with the ginseng root and its legendary prowess, the plant species was named *panax* derived from the Greek word *panakeia* or panacea, which means all-curing.

B) The Basic Chemistry of Ginseng

There are thousands of scientific studies from the United States, Russia, China, Korea, Japan and other smaller countries lauding the ability of ginseng to assist the body to better metabolize stress and balance its hormones, along with numerous other claims. The root of ginseng offers natural active ingredients. The most important are the saponins (ginsenosides). The complex carbohydrate molecules, or saponins, are especially helpful to the central nervous system and endocrine system. When analyzing the ginsenosides, research has been able to find the effects they have on different body systems. Chinese medicine often compartmentalizes treatments into a paradigm of having hot (*yang*) and or cold (*yin*) properties used for alleviating various aliments. Since ginseng is effective in maintaining balance by having ginsenosides that both stimulate and mitigate different body systems, its effects are conducive to the Chinese model that was developed thousands of years before modern lab tests could validate their theories with scientific explanations.

The amount of ginsenosides in each particular root can vary due to the health and location of the respective plant. The research shows that the Asian ginseng generally offers specimens with ginsenosides that stimulate the body, while the cultivated North American root tends to mollify an overactive system making the North American herb reputedly great for mitigating stress, reducing swollen prostate in men, and helping women with hormonal fluctuations during menopause. The claims of the miraculous delivered by this root are numerous stretching from shrinking tumors to growing hair, certainly we would caution investing credence into the more outlandish assertions. However science has proven the potentially salubrious effects on our health from this root in how it facilitates the ability of the body to cope with stress, balance hormone production, and increase strength as well as energy. The balancing of hormone production alone impacts many of the important functions of the human body including blood pressure, blood circulation, endurance, healing, and sleep

Unfortunately the roots that offer the highest quality and amounts of ginsenosides are the organic, older, and more rare wild roots. It can be six years before sufficient numbers of ginsenosides are produced and as much as two decades before the root produces its full range. The price for such aged roots or products comprised purely of them will be high compared to the bulk of products sold consisting of cultivated roots, or worse the ginseng impostors. Whether you subscribe to the studies extolling ginseng or not, consumers do, making this root a lucrative cash crop.

C) Types of Ginseng

You may read about other plants in the ginseng family being used in a variety of products and applications seemingly trying to capitalize on the ginseng name without large scale studies or research conducted to merit such use. Ginseng, the name, technically takes in a group of perennial herbs that are deciduous and are in the Araliaceae family. In recent decades the *panax* genus of this family as well as other branches have been commercially exploited, it is not to say that other *panax* or ginseng-family plants are entirely devoid of medicinal value but rather they are not proven to possess the healing potential and profit of Oriental or Asian ginseng (*panax ginseng*) and North American ginseng (*panax quinquefolium*) also commonly called American ginseng. The *panax ginseng* and *panax quinquefolium* are the plants that are attributed with having the vast range of healing properties and are thus in the greatest demand.

Although this book is essentially about successfully growing North American or *panax quinquefolium* it is wise to have a brief understanding of the other types of ginseng. Next is a sample of some of the ginsengs that you are likely to run across possibly in the wild or being offered for sale in the health food section of your local supermarket, herb store, or on the Internet. Take note that in May 2002 a congressional amendment to the Federal Food, Drug, and Cosmetic Act was signed into law stating that only products made with the genus *panax* can be referred to as *ginseng* on the labels or in the advertising of such items. However every product imported into, or certainly purchased outside of, the United States is impossible to regulate. Furthermore just being of the *panax* genus does not guarantee the herb used has the healing qualities of North American and Asian ginseng.

(i) American or North American Ginseng (*panax quinquefolium*)

(ii) Oriental Ginseng (*panax ginseng*)

(iii) Dwarf Ginseng (*panax trifolius*), and other lesser *panax* species

(iv) Siberian Ginseng (*eleutherococcus senticosus*)

(i) North American Ginseng is *panax quinquefolium.* If you are not familiar with Latin then that name likely seems long, but it roughly translates to five-leafleted plant. It is of the Araliaceae family where it is classified as an herbaceous perennial, or herb that comes up every year.

It is native to the Central region of North America. It can grow wild as far north as Manitoba, Quebec, or Ontario and as far south as Alabama, Oklahoma, Mississippi, and northern Georgia if the proper growing conditions are met. The natural range of the wild plant tends not to be further west than Minnesota, Missouri, or Arkansas while extending up most of the eastern United States from northern Georgia to Maine. North American ginseng can however be grown virtually in every state if the conditions exist or are created. The Pacific Northwest offers many ideal locations and growers even exist in Texas, Florida, and Arizona. The ideal habitat in the wild is under a primarily hardwood canopy on a northeastern slope with rich but well-drained loamy soil.

North American ginseng is smaller in size compared to its Asian cousin and is believed to be slightly different chemically but still shares the sought after medicinal qualities. The appearance of the plant may somewhat differ with the climate cosmetically and the berries may offer three seeds to a berry in the south as opposed to two seeds per berry in the north, nonetheless overall these are minor differences.

Its growing season is generally from May to September. The mature plants flower in June or July, then the greenish-white self-pollinating flowers develop into berries, which usually are ripe by late summer (more on the description of North American ginseng in *Section D* of this chapter).

(ii) Oriental Ginseng is *panax ginseng*. It is native to Eastern Asia where wild specimens have become extremely rare and only occasionally are still found. Nevertheless to meet demand massive cultivation operations presently flourish in Korea and China. The plant is very similar to its North American counterpart in physical appearance with only slight variations (such as a more slender leaf and a plant that is slightly larger in stature).

Three terms to describe the processed Asian or Oriental ginseng that you may encounter in commercial products are: *Red Ginseng* (Chinese), *White Cultivated Ginseng*, and *Yi Sun Ginseng*. Briefly explained they are all grown by human production. The *White Cultivated Ginseng* is the root prior to processing. In the drying process herbs used during drying give the root a red hue creating *Red Ginseng*, this is sometimes named from the province it was grown in e.g. *Manchurian Red Ginseng*. *Yi Sun Ginseng* is very expensive because although cultivated, it is grown in woodlands simulating wild ginseng. Also note that Korean ginseng although oriental, may have inferior healing properties because of the practice of removing the outer skin of the root prior to processing. This skin contains most of the ginsenosides. Also of the Asian countries and their ginseng, the Japanese ginseng is alleged to be one of the worst, offering a poor quality root.

(iii) Dwarf Ginseng is *panax trifolium*. This is a small less valuable member of the ginseng family. The root more resembles an onion ball than the traditional North American or Oriental ginseng root. There is a growing market for its sale but presently more because of it sharing the ginseng namesake than any other reason. It grows naturally in North America and is believed by herbalists to contain some limited medicinal qualities but nothing compared to Oriental and North American ginseng. Be watchful of cheap *panax* species like *trifolium* being used in commercial products exploiting the scientifically documented benefits of Oriental and North American ginseng.

Even Asian countries are trying to capitalize on the *panax* name and other significantly lesser quality plants of the ginseng family. They are pushed to the unwary and should be avoided. Some examples are: *Chu-Chieh Seng, San-Chi, Japonicus*, and *NotoGinseng*. If you read these as the ginseng in a product you are taking or considering purchasing, it should scream red herring at you, they are using a *panax* herb but that is it. Be watchful of companies and herbalists that sell these products along side of similarly priced Oriental and North American ginseng.

(iv) Siberian Ginseng, or properly labeled Eleuthero,
is *eleutherococcus senticosus*.

Siberian ginseng (Eleuthero) is characterized as a thorny shrub plant with deep green compound leaves that feature five leaflets. To some extent these compound leaves resemble the compound leaves of North American and Asian ginseng. A vigorous grower and more tolerant to sunlight, it can reach heights of eight feet in seven years. (*see* Ginseng Picture #1).

This herb is a distant relative to the ginseng family but is not of the *panax* species and in fact is in a completely different genus. The common comparison is that it is as related to North American ginseng as humans are to the monkey. In fact it falls in an unfortunate category of other herbs that have "ginseng" in their name for reasons of commercial convenience rather than botanical merit. To the credit of Siberian ginseng it has been extensively studied by the Russian government and found to offer medicinal qualities similar in some respects to Asian ginseng especially as a stimulant with adaptogenic qualities. Adaptogenic means that it encourages the body to adapt to external stress caused by illness and injury. It also has been used in experimental HIV treatments.

Native to the northeastern section of Asia, it grows in present day China, Korea, and Russia. Also with vast amounts in what was the former Soviet Union, numerous studies were

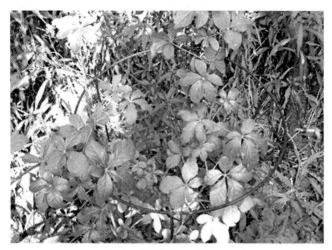

Siberian Ginseng (above)

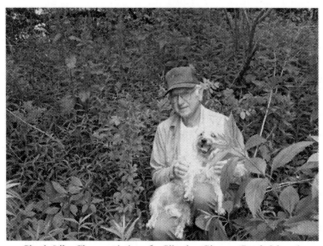

Shrub-Like Characteristics of a Siberian Ginseng Patch (above)

administered to evaluate its ability as a medicinal herb by the Soviet government. The test subjects in the studies did not show adverse side effects while demonstrating positive results after consuming the herb for two months. Siberian ginseng was found to offer noticeable adaptogenic properties along with over thirty compounds responsible for its efficacy in aiding the body to perform efficiently under stress. Furthermore it has been and is used by millions of Russians ranging from the average citizen to professional/Olympic athletes and cosmonauts. Also Chinese herbalists have been using this root for over 2,000 years, where it is still used today. Despite its potential, it remains a great deal cheaper than the Asian and North American root, unless you are buying it in the form of partially overpriced supplements. Currently production of Siberian ginseng in America is limited but seeds and plants can be purchased at a handful of stores for those that want to dabble (*see* Appendix).

Once again like Siberian ginseng, companies cannot resist attaching the "ginseng" name to hawk their products even if they are completely devoid of the constituent chemicals of the valuable North American and Asian *panax* roots. Notwithstanding it being prohibited to label non-*panax* herbs as ginseng here is a sample of some spuriously named "ginsengs" to avoid: *Wild Red American Ginseng* (not to be confused with *Chinese Red Ginseng* discussed earlier), *Wild Red Desert Ginseng*, derived from the plant Canaigre; *South American Ginseng*, or *Brazilian Ginseng*, derived from the Suma plant containing some adaptogenic qualities; and *Ayurvedic Ginseng* from the Aschwiganda plant of India. It is likely these plants can help the body in some way, but not in the manner that the true Asian and North American ginseng have scientifically been proven to do. Marketers will invariably *create* more *ginsengs* as demand and interest grows in this herb. They will also likely stretch the claims of the lower quality *panax* herbs to be able to legally assert a product has ginseng as a component at a cheaper cost to them, however now you will not be duped by such attempts.

D) Characteristics of North American Ginseng

The thrust of this field manual is to concentrate on growing and identifying North American ginseng. At first it may resemble other plants in the woods but after careful observation and study of its appearance, you should have little difficulty identifying it. Throughout this section refer to the Ginseng Diagram to familiarize yourself with the various parts of the ginseng plant.

(i) Appearance and Plant Structure

Ginseng requires a climate that receives at least ½ an inch of rain per week on average but the safe range is 20 – 30 inches of annual rainfall. It garners some protection by blending with its neighboring green leafy plants growing in the woods during the summer months and dying back during the fall. Other plants that like to grow in suitable forest conditions or near ginseng, and may even slightly resemble it, are referred to as companion plants. Sometimes ginseng will even be growing among a cluster of these companion plants. The most popular include: bloodroot, black and blue cohosh, goldenseal, Christmas fern, baneberry, Dutchman's pipe, spicebush, maidenhair fern, wild ginger, wild sarsaparilla, Indian turnip, and jack-in-the-pulpit. Ginseng does not have to be growing with them but companion plants can indicate certain conditions precedent have been established for ginseng to be present. Also ginseng in its natural state will likely be growing under deciduous hardwoods such as: hickory, basswood, elm, ash, walnut, maple and oak. One of the most common shade trees for ginseng in the North is the sugar maple while in the South it is the tulip poplar.

The financially valuable part of the ginseng plant is its root nonetheless it is the plant itself that will be the most important while it is growing, and a plant that you will need to recognize. Ginseng is likely to be growing on a north or northeast-facing slope under a hardwood forest that offers around 70 – 80 percent shade and a humus-rich, well-drained soil, that has a pH between 3.8 – 7.1 (although the fringe numbers on this scale are far from ideal, ginseng prefers a pH of 5.5 – 6.5). During the growing season extending from May through to September healthy ginseng has greenish stems with a slight trace of purple, and offers green leaflets until the fall when the leaves turn yellowish-light green and die back for the year. The mature plants, usually at least three years of age (but sometimes two year old plants), will offer up a round flower group in June or July containing small white and green flowers. These flowers contain both the stamen and carpel and thus are equipped for self-pollination.

During the summer growing season a small bud will develop on the top of the ginseng root adjacent to the stalk of the plant, this will be where the plant emerges next year. By August, the berries, (about the size of two kernels of sweet corn fused together), remain green until the middle of the month and early September. The berries in the cluster then turn crimson red while the once green leaves of the plant begin to turn their yellowish/light green thus signaling the end of the growing season.

After the top dies back, the root will slightly contract and shrink down into the soil to protect the bud for next year, which remains attached to the top of the root.

Years of this contracting, creates rings horizontally covering the exterior of a mature root giving it almost the ribbed look of a Slinky on its exterior. These rings can greatly add to the value of a wild and woods-simulated root showing a potential buyer that they are buying a good quality and aged root as opposed to the field cultivated roots, which generally lack this natural ringed-look.

Refer to the Ginseng Diagram

(i) Root Rings   (iv) Fork   (vii) Compound Leaf
(ii) Stem/Plant Stalk   (v) Leaf Stalk (viii) Flower/Berry/Seed Cluster
(iii)Bud   (vi) Leaflets

(ii) Physical Development
Ginseng stands from as low as one inch to over 1½ feet tall depending on its age and health. A healthy plant will alter its appearance during the first several growing seasons, the most extreme being the first 1 - 4 years. Since the plant changes as

it matures you must acquaint yourself with its growing cycle. Next is an ideal growth model for a wild plant that survives against the piteous odds nature grants it (*see* Ginseng Picture Group #2). Once the wild plant begins to mature its physical development should also mirror the growth of woods-grown and woods-cultivated ginseng.

From Seed: The Amazing Journey

First a ripe red berry (containing 1 - 3 seeds) falls from the seed cluster of a plant to the ground at the end of the growing season during late August or September.

At this point the berry pulp around the seeds provides a natural protection as the berry lays still or tumbles along the forest floor by way of weathering until it lodges near a rock, tree trunk, natural indentation, or is consumed and passed through the digestive system of an animal. The leaves from the trees soon fall covering the forest floor providing a natural blanket of mulch for the adventurous berry.

The berry pulp-protection gives way to decomposition and the seeds remain for 19 - 21 months under the leaves and any subsequent mulch-protection that covers them. The seeds wait during their natural stratification process until they are ready to germinate.

After sitting out the first year, the yearling ginseng plant, will produce its first green plant top over a year and a half from when it fell as a berry. For the seed's second year and first growing year, it will be a humble plant. A single green stem will grow, with one compound leaf comprised of three ovate shaped leaflets having serrated edges and tips that slowly taper to a blunt point. Each leaflet is about 1 - 1½-inches in length, resembling a strawberry plant. Ginseng is exceedingly vulnerable during this first growing year. During this season it will also have created its rhizome bud for next year. The root size by the fall will be about ½ - 1 inch long and ¼ of an inch in width.

In subsequent growing seasons the plant will usually add leaf stalks and leaf clusters of leaflets. Generally after the first year of growth the ginseng plant begins to more resemble its classic look. The development of further plant growth differs due to the environment and other variables. It is believed that the growth of the above ground plant is predicated on root development and size as well as overall health. The maturity and growth of the ginseng plant can often be grouped into the following paradigm.

Two-Year Old Plants

Usually one prong emerges from the main stalk with five leaflets, or two sets of leaves with only three leaflets or a combination thereof. Occasionally it will send up a similar looking plant as its first year with only three leaflets if it did poorly the first year or, just as rare, if it really thrived it my send up two full leaves, each leaf comprising five leaflets and a berry cluster. Although in the second growing season the plant can develop a second leaf stalk, usually look for one, and the leaflets will often be in clusters of five instead of the three from the first year. Notice the leaflets generally feature three larger and two smaller sizes per compound leaf and are shaped as oblanceolate mixed with ovate, whereas the leaflets are wider at the top than the bottom but taper to a point like the top half of the ovate leaflets and featuring serrated edges.

Three to Seven-Year Old Plants

During the third growing season there will be a second or third leaf stalk growing from the plant stalk forking out at a single junction. Also aside from these leaf stalks an additional protruding stalk producing a cluster of tiny green and white flowers may appear. All leaf and berry stalks will fork from a central point on the plant. The flowers will turn to green berries and by late summer (or early fall) will be ready to harvest when the berries take on a red color.

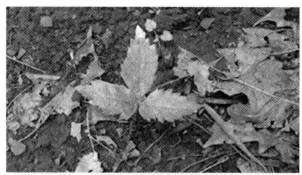

Ginseng Yearling (above)

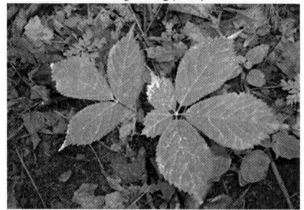

Leaflet Variations of Ginseng in its 2nd Year of Growth (above &below)

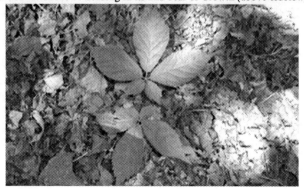

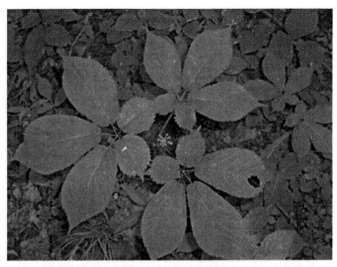

*Mature 3-Pronged Ginseng Plant with Minor Insect
damage on leaflet (above)*

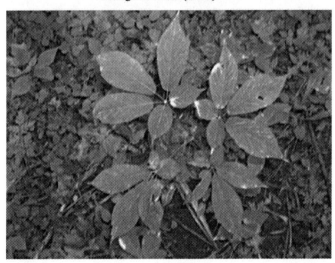

Mature 4-Pronged Ginseng Plant With Spray Residue on Leaflets (above)

By the fourth growing season ginseng usually takes on
the conventional look of a mature plant. The plant may grow
a fourth leaf stalk as well as a larger berry cluster and it may

reach as high as eighteen inches or more under ideal conditions. Generally there will be three stalks present and a berry cluster offering 30 – 50 berries. With good health and maturity a plant will develop a fourth stalk and if left to grow even a fifth stalk, again it is seemingly root size and health that determines the amount of stalks more than age.

(iii) The Age of a Root

Establishing the age of the plant comes from counting the bumps on the top of a protruding gnarled part of the root. These are called the neck scars. They are formed when ginseng produces its bud for the next growing season while in the middle of the present one. During July when the small bud grows up from the root, in the opposite direction but adjacent to the plant stalk (*see* Ginseng Diagram) it leaves what is referred to as a scar. This scarring is not the most accurate way to deduce the age of a root, as sometimes the neck scarring can be damaged in its habitat or a root can even go dormant for one or even two years thus potentially skewing the ability to accurately ascribe an age to a wild ginseng root. If a root decides to remain dormant there will not be any new buds created for that year, researchers are not sure why ginseng does this. Possibly it is a self-defense reaction when the root does not feel it has the adequate energy to offer up a healthy plant in a given growing season.

Ginseng Tip!

The leaves and leaflets extend out from a common point similar to blades on an airplane propeller. This is a quick way to visually separate potential ginseng from similar looking companion plants such as wild sarsaparilla. Also mutations and variations occur in nature from plant size, seed yielding ability, and strength, the prior descriptions provided are for the average plant that you will grow or find in the woods.

Chapter II

Growing Ginseng

A) The Growing Methods

There are essentially four methods in which ginseng grows or is grown. The cardinal rule requiring adequate **SDS (Shade, Drainage, Soil)** applies. The classifications of ginseng for this purpose are:
   (i) Wild
   (ii) Wild-Simulated
   (iii) Woods-Grown
   (iv) Field Cultivated or Commercially Grown

(i) Wild

Wild root has become scarce over the years due to greedy exploitation and in the more disturbing cases abject carelessness in stewardship of this plant. Of the four classifications, wild demands the highest price thus spurring ginseng poachers and hunters to comb the areas they believe it tends to naturally be growing during the late summer and early fall. The plant itself prefers rich forest soil with excellent drainage, a soil pH between 5.5 – 6.5 and 70 percent shade in an overhead hardwood canopy. As discussed earlier, the pH can be much lower and higher, but the 5.5 – 6.5 range is ideal. Also direct sunlight or overexposure of sun will inhibit or destroy ginseng, which is why it prefers a northeastern-facing sloped hill. It may be growing from the forest floor in many places, realizing that before it was a plant it was a seed that likely tumbled or was discharged. Natural soil shelves on a sloped hill, near a large rock, or very close to the base of a tree offer great spots. Also steep riverbanks, ravines, and mountainous outcrops can yield wild specimens.

The pH may only be 3.8, the hillside may face the south instead of the favored northeastern side, there may even be some pine trees growing near wild plants souring the soil. However ginseng will only grow where there is adequate **shade**, **drainage**, and good **soil**, thus likely on a topographical slope of some degree preferring a porous but nutritious soil (limestone ridges are great). Therefore although ginseng will grow in other than ideal areas, now you can winnow through where it will not be such as: clearings, open fields, pastures, swamps, creek beds, and grass thickets.

For traditionally wild plants to be occupying an area it likely has to be a section of forest that was not clear-cut during the last century, used as pastures, or logged thin. Luckily for wild ginseng the rough-terrain-woods it prefers have often been left alone since colonial times only because it could not be easily used by settlers. As for recently undisturbed hardwood-reclaimed areas that offer the shade, pH, and drainage that ginseng prefers, nature does auspiciously allow for the occasional seed broadcast through bird or other animal droppings to propagate new populations. However the odds are capriciously against ginseng to succeed without help so always harvest responsibly and duly according to applicable state and federal laws. This involves but is not limited to harvesting during the proper time, usually late summer or early fall, a commencement date that changes from state to state. Also you must pick only mature plants (at least 10 years of age), and carefully planting its berries within 50 feet of where the plant was growing, as federal regulations require. The berries should then be promptly planted about ¼ - ½ inch deep and then covered with an additional ¼ inch of crumpled decayed leaves as mulch.

Wild plants have become so rare that we will not harvest them unless they are in danger of being destroyed. Threats such as development, logging, or even in rare cases potential disease due to over population are suitable justifications to duly remove and replant them in the fall. There are many hunters who justify plucking a single stark living specimen from an area with the argument that like hardwood lumber, ginseng is a woodland crop that needs to be harvested. However this is balderdash. These roots if left unmolested can live three decades and even a root exceeding 100 years of age was found in the early 1980s in China. Suitable discretion should be employed with the extraction of wild roots. Furthermore ginseng is sold as dry root and it requires 100 - 300 roots, depending on their size, for just one pound. This means to achieve a dry pound a hunter could easily devastate a sparse local population of ginseng in just one weekend afternoon.

Advantages: Although treasured and rare substantial numbers of roots are out there in North America unlike Asia. In West Virginia alone the estimates by the state put the number in 2004 at 95 million plants growing. As of the late 1990s and early 2000s the United States was exporting over 31,000,000 wild plants annually. All you need is the expertise, free time, the legal right, the property, and some digging implements.

Disadvantages: First wild ginseng is covered under the Convention on International Trade in Endangered Species of Wild Fauna and Flora, Appendix II, because of its threatened status. Under this, the U.S. Federal Fish and Wildlife Service call upon the states to regulate and monitor the sale and export of wild ginseng. Unlawful harvesting may earn a poacher a criminal record and fines, unfortunately the National Park Service has discovered the existence of a lucrative black market where wild roots harvested on protected lands, such as national parks, is also destroying what should otherwise be safe populations.
Furthermore beginning in the harvest season of 2005 the U.S. Fish and Wildlife Service restricted the exportation of wild roots that were less than 10 years old. Prior to this 2005 regulation the wild root only had to be five years of age, adding extra importance to the careful extraction of roots allowing for full preservation

of the neck scars. Since this regulation was foisted on ginseng hunters late in 2005 there was a one-year period where roots of the previously acceptable age of five years (and those up to 10 years of age) could still be sold. This is a problematic rule and it will likely spur an already expanding black market because once in the Far East, where most of the American wild root is exported, whether the age of a root is 10 years or five years it will not dissuade Asian buyers once the root is there. Should you dig a ginseng plant and find that the root can only demonstrate neck scars for nine years or less then properly and immediately replant the root.

Assuming a hunter is lawfully harvesting wild ginseng they must acquaint themselves with both applicable state and federal laws and regulations. Some states have even adopted stricter regulations, Maine has listed ginseng as endangered and Michigan has already labeled it threatened. Also states offer differing dates from when the legal season begins. Ginseng is not only protected by the law sometimes it is protected by nature while growing in dangerous places. Especially if you live in the South be aware of poisonous snakes, or other unfriendly animals. You may need to obtain permission to collect roots if you do not own suitable land. The hunt may take you on quite a journey, be sure you are prepared with adequate provisions, protection, and again always harvest responsibly.

(ii) Wild-Simulated

This method of raising ginseng requires the grower to own or have legal access to use or rent vast areas of suitable land. The goal is to replicate the plant in its wild habitat in woodlands that may have been suitable for wild ginseng had nature granted the opportunity. By replicating the natural development you plant the seeds (green or stratified seed is discussed later in Chapter V) or plant root-stock as it is found in nature. This means sowing it in the suitable environs of the wild (covered earlier) and spaced in small clusters of 1 - 2 per square foot. With wild-simulated you have the advantage of picking the best places, unlike nature. Spraying frequency and fertilizing depends on the discretion of the grower. The degree of spraying ranges from occasional and may include only giving the plant-patches a douse of fungicide. However to properly simulate the wild, the plants should be left to their own accord. Keeping in mind if a grower wants to tinker with the plants in any significant degree they may actually be creating a woods-grown crop.

Advantages: Wild-Simulated offers the easiest startup. Your initial investment can be as little as a pound of stratified seed or several hundred young ginseng roots (known as rootlets), a garden trowel or hand-held rake, and some free time in the woods. Depending on where you purchase your seeds a pound of stratified can cost between $55 - $100 for an amount between 6,500 to as many as 8,500 seeds, because seed size slightly differs so does the amount in each pound. You will not need to spend nearly as much time and money on supplies especially regarding the spray chemicals as larger cultivators have to. The idea is for the woods-simulated growers to "simulate" wild ginseng by being largely organic. Never use human or animal manure to fertilize despite its organic qualities, animal fertilizer risks imbuing the root with a dung-flavor and human manure has a host of problems.

Although some do occasionally spray fungicides, the crop is supposed to be left natural. This is part of the reason why wild-simulated currently can bring nearly thrice what the heavily fertilized field cultivated ginseng sells for. Also the organic food market is a $7.8 billion industry annually and expanding every year, with a successfully grown wild-simulated crop and effective marketing to gourmet markets, the potential for success is only limited by your ability to plant it and passively keep it alive.

Wild-simulated ginseng is planted in isolated clusters, should vermin or disease strike, the characteristics that help contain it in nature will apply. However it is never wise to let disease run rampant regardless of the growing technique you employ, non-chemical precautions such as removing and either carefully discarding or safely quarantining sick plants is a must. Wild-simulated also does not need a seedbed because you plant the seeds where they remain, or close by a parent plant. As the grower, your role theoretically ends once the seed is planted. It is wise to gather the berries that will be produced in subsequent years and properly plant them. Letting animals feed on the berries helps let them naturally spread which is altruistic, however the crimson red berries act as a calling card to wild animals that may also dig at the root and humans who will likewise do the same. An inconspicuous ginseng plant is a much safer plant.

Method

Once the suitable location on the forest floor is found, prepare the ground. Loosen up the soil with your garden trowel (or if a large area is planned a rented or owned rototiller is ideal) to a depth of 6 - 8 inches. Just before planting seeds or rootlets it is always ideal to disinfect them (*see* Chapter V Seed, Section D). If you are going totally organic this step can be omitted. For regular growers mix a 1-tablespoon bleach to 1-gallon water solution and soak the seeds for eight minutes, then thoroughly rinse with water. However a better choice is to apply a 1-tablespoon fungicide to 1-gallon water mixture with a ginseng fungicide like Manzate 200 then soak the seeds for several minutes and rinse them with clean water. Either disinfecting method employed should clean the seeds or rootlets. The bleach is likely going to kill some seed but a fungus on the seed can kill far more in time, remember the better choice is to use a commercial ginseng fungicide mixture made from Manzate if it can be readily obtained.

Then plant the stratified ginseng seed about ½ - 1 inch below the surface, if the soil is very loose sow the seed between ¾ - 1 inch, if it is dense than ½ - ¾ of an inch deep. If you begin with rootlets then plant them so that their buds are only ½ - 1 inch below the surface. Green seed is not recommended, however if used, plant it no more than ½ inch below the surface since it will be sitting another year before growth. Space the rootlets or seed at least 8 - 10 inches apart, keeping in mind that in the wild one or two plants per square foot is best. Cover the seed or fill the soil in around the rootlet and then look for some decayed leaves to act as mulch to place over the area. Break the dried leaves up in your hands and cover the crop. Ideally at least ¾ - 1 inch of mulch is used, but since this is woods-simulated a modest covering of ½ - ¾ inch should suffice in most climates.

Shade

The trees of the forest provide for your natural canopy of shade, be sure to periodically check throughout the day to be confident the sunlight is indirect, and that the area is receiving at least 70 percent shade. Observe where the rays of sunlight pierce the canopy, flag those areas with a marker and avoid them. Also take notice of forest ground that already has plants that enjoy increased sun such as grasses, this should indicate where potential holes are in the forest canopy. As with wild ginseng, ideally you will plant wild-simulated under a cover that includes some of the traditionally preferred deciduous hardwood trees this list includes: basswood, elm, ash, hickory, red oak, sugar maple, white oak, and walnut. Note that if your soil is already on the acidic end of the scale, too much oak may make the soil too sour, also make sure you are not too dependent on any elm trees in your shade as they might succumb to disease, however the presence of elm is a good indication of satisfactory soil drainage. After you locate an ideal planting area make one more consideration, preferably choose an area that will not be disturbed due to logging, residential development, or other activity in the foreseeable future.

Drainage

Test the potential drainage of your desired area by looking at the slope of the land, there needs to be at least a minimal degree of grade to the ground allowing for the dispersal of surface water. For this reason choose the higher portion of a hillside avoiding areas that may become submerged after winter melt-off or heavy rainstorms. Again look to plants already growing in the potential area for soil compatibility, however companion plants like jack-in-the-pulpit, nettles, mayapple and some ferns tolerate far more sunlight than ginseng can, they imply suitable soil nutrients present but not necessarily adequate shade.

Fungi will quickly assail the ginseng root if it is too wet. The soil should be moist to the touch but not wet and sticky. It is best to check the potential area after heavy rains and before planting to assess its viability as a site. If drainage is your only problem to an otherwise perfect site, experiment with making a trench with garden implements or a rototiller to bypass sporadic streams of runoff.

Soil

The existing ground and soil is your garden. Therefore only minor adulterations should be made. We have found wild ginseng patches in soil with a pH of only 3.7 nearly 2.0 less than the preferred range thus the importance of pH weighs in on not so much the ability of ginseng to survive but on its ability to thrive and fight disease. For this reason test the soil of the potential site with a simple soil testing kit or inexpensive soil meter and try avoiding the trees that facilitate sour soil conditions such as pine (and most coniferous) or large amounts of oak. If you are lacking the ideal growing site remember that people have been successful growing ginseng under a canopy with some pines and the soil can always be altered to some degree with amendments, as described in the next chapter. However whenever you deviate from the preferred paradigm of ideal **SDS**, results vary. We know ginseng prefers moist, rich, loamy, dark, well-drained forest soil, but if your land does not offer this then experiment with woods-simulated and try to see if you can create a viable environment before you invest heavily in woods-grown.

Disadvantages: Though an excellent and inexpensive manner to experiment with growing ginseng, with wild-simulated your crop will likely be modest. Even if you own or have legal access to hundreds of acres of land, finding ideal preexisting natural locations may present a challenge. Planting seed sparse can take a long time to complete and germination of seed and subsequent plant success may only be 30 – 40 percent after eight years even with ideal growing conditions.

Before harvesting, these plants have to survive perhaps 7 - 10 years before your roots are a suitable size to extract. This is because they tend to grow slow like the wild plants unless they are fertilized. If conservatively fertilized with some luck you might be able to harvest in 5 – 6 years but remember too much fertilizing will give the root a less valuable commercial-look and may make your plants more vulnerable to disease. If you leave them to nature they may be smaller but will look more akin to the desired wild ginseng in regard to color, shape, and size, also remember that on average 100 - 300 dried roots are needed to make a pound. Unless you are fortunate with your attempts it will not likely bring in a substantial income. Finally the 2005 regulation demanding that all wild root harvested for export must be at least 10 years of age prevents wild-simulated growers from being able to sell roots younger than 10 years for the price of wild, as they could in theory before this change.

(iii) Woods-Grown

This is ginseng grown in large gardens and patches in the natural setting of the forest. Pesticides and fungicides are employed but with far less frequency than in field cultivation beds under artificial shade. Woods-grown is the most efficient way a landowner can utilize the natural habitat of their woodland while producing substantial crops. There is a sliding scale as some growers may plant their crops closer and spray more resembling commercial field cultivation while others plant sparse and spray less more resembling wild-simulated. The grower must

employ what is most suitable for them. This depends on their
expectations, resources, and the land they have to work with.

Advantages: If you are a landowner living with several acres
of woodland this can be a profitable hobby, especially if you
already have the basic equipment and machinery available from
other pursuits. This method yields a crop with higher marketable
value than field cultivated and without the tremendous expense
of building the artificial shade they need to employ. The yield is
usually greater than wild-simulated because it is easier to care for
the plants, and more survive with regular spraying. Ginseng has
many enemies ready to attack thwarting its development ranging
from slugs, disease, poachers, deer, voles, and mice to name a
few. With woods-grown ginseng, while your crop enjoys the
natural habitat of growing in the wild, it has you as its sentinel
to reduce the high rate of attrition experienced in nature from
these aforementioned enemies.

By creating this cash crop you are helping the environment,
even though you will harvest most of your berries some will be
invariably consumed by animals reintroducing ginseng to your
area. Also clearing the undergrowth in the woods is healthier
for your woodlands. Once your gardens are created and seeds
or plants are planted, the upkeep of spraying on average every
10 – 14 days during the summer growing season is minimal.
Furthermore after the ginseng is harvested from your gardens,
with the gardens already being created, the space can be utilized
to grow goldenseal. It is never a good idea to replant ginseng
in the same plot after it has been harvested, it is not done with
the field cultivated technique because the soil will not allow
another crop. This possibly is due to the inundation of additives,
chemicals, and accumulated toxins during the four years of
growth. This would not in and of itself preclude woods-grown
growers since far less chemicals and concentrations of plants
occupy each square foot of garden nonetheless it is best to move
to a new area if you can as our yields have been drastically less

from recycled gardens. Goldenseal is an ideal secondary cash crop suited for this purpose, which is covered in Chapter IX Growing Goldenseal.

Method

The first step is to look to the wisdom of nature. If you have not personally witnessed this herb growing in the wild, from this manual you now know where it might grow and certainly where it will not. Ideally plan your potential ginseng gardens during the winter, having first carried out your **SDS** assessment of available land (with good shade), drainage, and soil from the previous fall. Now you can sort through the ideal places on your property. If you are anxious to get started everything can be done in the spring before May but be aware your window for planning, preparing, and planting may be short in the spring compared to the following fall.

Shade

As learned from the sections on wild growing and wild-simulated ginseng, proper shade is paramount. With woods-grown the existing trees are your canopy. Ginseng prefers growing under hardwoods like basswood, hickory, iron wood, ash, sugar maple, elm, and oak, however the most important aspect to consider is if the foliage creates enough natural shade. Walk through your woods during the day in the summer, take notes and mark where direct sunlight permeates for long periods. These are places you will seek to avoid. Usually they are small pockets that can easily be worked around, remember you want indirect sunlight resulting in 70 - 80 percent shade. Excessive pine and oak trees may make your soil too sour but that may be augmented with amendments to some degree, which is explained later.

Take stock of what trees comprise your shade canopy and ask yourself, are they healthy? For instance given the Dutch elm disease you would never want to plant under elm and be compelled to depend on them for your shade in case they die, or a moribund tree that will force you to build extra shade if it falls apart. Watch for damaged limbs that can fall onto your garden, and onto plants. Planting under mature trees is ideal, because you can clear out the lower limbs and brush as this allows good airflow, which helps moderate temperatures and mitigate disease. Ginseng does not like to be too warm, proper airflow helps reduce this heat and discourages fungi growth.

Make sure your trees produce leaves at the right time. Long ago we once prepared beds and planted over 18,000 seeds under a full canopy that featured predominately ash, only to realize the following spring that the ginseng plants were peeking out of the ground (during the third week of May) weeks before the ash leaves were developed enough to provide adequate protection. The verdant foliage was near complete on every hardwood except those ash trees. At that point we were forced to build ersatz artificial-shade. Then later in that summer we noticed that those same ash trees also lost their leaves earlier than the other hardwoods luckily by then the growing season for ginseng had for the most part ceased. Another shade tree to watch for is the black locust, they also are late to produce their leaves. These are simple things you may not notice just casually looking at your hardwood trees season to season from your house, because normally a couple weeks difference on leaf development does not matter unless you are planting ginseng and depending on that shade. Therefore it is well worth your time to place adequate energy into preparation and analysis before preparing the gardens and sowing seed. You do not need a degree in botany or forestry just a keen eye, a notebook, and a willingness to observe and learn.

If you own woodland that is too dense you may have to remove some trees. What is too dense? The high end of shade that can be tolerated is around 85 percent, this is an easy number to write but difficult to quantify in meaningful terms. At this point exercise prudent judgment. Remember that ginseng prefers all the light that it can withstand, so analyze your trees, look for companion plants, and if it is so dark and dense that you cannot tell if it is a sunny or cloudy sky while beneath them, then consider doing some clearing. When contemplating these plots and the potential shade bearing trees they will be under, you also do not want to create beds where there will be a harvesting of lumber or firewood while the plants are growing. You are looking for an area of woods that can remain relatively undisturbed for the next 5 – 7 years despite routine maintenance. In the event that shade trees are destroyed by nature through weather or disease you can construct shade or transplant the ginseng, however you want to save transplanting as a last resort since it can be a dark art and a trap for the novice.

A note about maple, in many ways it is an ideal tree. Usually maple creates a strong, healthy, and full tree, but its roots under the soil can grow into a thick fibrous mess invading your gardens and creating problems when you harvest the ginseng. Sometimes you are simply forced to work with what you have but if planting under a predominately maple canopy then be aware of this potential problem.

Drainage

Ginseng does not grow well where there is poor drainage. The root can quickly give way to root-rot and other fungi. It can be tantalizing while on your own trying to sort out what is the preferred moist soil condition compared to what is considered too wet. As discussed with wild-simulated, if after tilling the soil (assuming this is done during a normal weather pattern), it is gummy to the touch, then it likely is too wet and devoid of the proper draining attributes. Remember that ginseng can fair far better in "drier" soil than "wetter than preferred" soil.

Northeastern slops are ideal due to the mitigated amount of direct sunlight usually received on them however your land will likely face different directions and may only offer a slight grade. In such a case, as long as shade is present, a slight grade can be improvised into a viable garden by using a rototiller. When preparing your garden simply create a raised or domed garden with a trench, it is easier than it may initially sound and is explained in Chapter IV.

Unlike wild-simulated, with woods-grown you have the opportunity while tilling large tracks of soil for your gardens to add leaf-mulch or even better hardwood sawdust (avoid oak).

When planning your beds give them a width of about four feet and create them so that they run or zig-zag down the sloping hillside like the nose of a human face as opposed to being terraced like the mouth on a face. This creates better drainage. Also trench the border of your garden with a parallel ditch running on the outside with the cultivator on your rototiller. This gives water a place to run should there be a cloud burst, heavy rain storm, or large amounts of melting snow. This is covered in full detail in Chapter IV Creating Gardens.

Soil

Sticking to our **SDS** formula after locating an area with adequate shade, good or at least suitable drainage, now you must carry out some soil testing. Check the pH with a kit or meter, make sure your soil is between 5.5 – 6.5 for suitable garden plots. After tilling to a depth of 6 – 8 inches you are given on excellent opportunity to really inspect the soil of the potential plot. Since, dark, rich, loamy, loose soil, filled with leaf mold is preferred, further leaf mold can be rototilled in before planting if your soil lacks the desired consistency. Avoid areas with clay filled soil offering poor drainage.

Disadvantages: Unless you are already engaged in some type of agricultural or horticultural pursuit, you will need to buy some machinery and supplies. The following are highly recommended: rototiller (rear tined and at least four horsepower), leaf vacuum, brush pruners, chainsaw, standard garden implements, backpack sprayer, fungicides & slug poison, and mulch.

After supplies your next investment is time. Woods-grown ginseng is often given small amounts of fertilizer and it likely will grow quicker than woods-simulated, but with smaller roots than field cultivated. Ginseng takes years (at least 4 – 5 growing years minimum) to reach a marketable and mature age, and you may need to wait 7 - 8 years to get a suitable size on your roots. Also time spent in the garden may need to be balanced with full time work, everyday obligations, and hopefully an understanding or cooperating family.

Preparing gardens can be very physical work, depending on how thick your woodlands are. If you have not been involved in physical activity either at work or through recreation it would not be a bad idea to have your doctor or a health professional give you a check-up. Preparing and maintaining ginseng gardens needs to be a labor of love. Pace yourself because it can be exhausting if you take on too much too quickly. Be realistic with your planning on how many beds you decide to create and do your homework on what areas will take more time to clear.

Spraying may be considered a disadvantage, it will need to be undertaken on a regular schedule because unlike wild-simulated you will have beds with thousands of plants growing only 6 – 8 inches apart and disease spreads quickly and easily, this is discussed in more detail in the Chapter VI Threats and Risk Management.

(iv) Field Cultivated

This is ginseng grown under artificial shade with plants packed in close proximity, with as many as 25 plants per square foot. Thus these crops receive high amounts of chemical sprays to prevent disease. They also are heavily fertilized. In theory these gardens could almost be established anywhere even your back lawn because the **SDS** paradigm is created by the grower. After each harvest you need more land, you never plant in gardens that have already yielded a crop. The soil builds up an intolerance to allow another commercial crop in the same plot.

Thus commercial operations move their gardens when finished with the land. Most commercial ginseng finding its way into the stream of commerce is grown in this manner.

Due to corporations and funding by governments in other countries to their respective growers the market price for this class of ginseng has continued to drop consistently. Canada has expanded its crops with well over 3,000 acres of field cultivated ginseng in the past two decades mainly in Ontario as well as British Columbia and even China is now growing hundreds of acres of North American ginseng in this manner. Each field cultivated acre is capable of yielding 2,000 pounds of ginseng. Therefore the price has fallen sharply, fluctuating, but presently ranging from $10-$25 per pound.

At first the idea of harvesting 2,000 pounds per acre in only 4 - 5 years (although some cultivators even turn out roots in three years) with a ready market might sound alluring. However the price of the materials needed to create the gardens and artificial shade has risen, especially the cost of lumber while prices paid for ginseng at auction have steadily dropped. The only time it would be logical for the average person to attempt to grow field cultivated ginseng under artificial shade is if you have a very small place on your property to experiment with just as a hobby or have a large amount of capital you want to play with and invest into the endeavor. Otherwise the large financial returns simply are not there as they were just ten years ago.

Advantages: The math speaks, 2,000 pounds selling for the conservative estimate of $12 a pound = $24,000 in 4 - 5 years, with four acres (4 x $24,000) would be $96,000 of gross profits. If you have access to wood then you can build your wooden shade similar to the lattice used on porches at a reduced price. Some growers sell their berries harvested from the plants for extra income but others remove the flower stalk early right after it emerges to give the root extra strength and growth. Either way the potential for profit is real.

Method

You can create the garden from a field or open space, if the area is flat be sure to create a raised bed and build artificial shade tall enough so that you can work underneath it, especially in regard to spraying.

Spraying is intensive. With plants fertilized and densely packed under artificial shade the opportunity and conditions for disease must be aggressively assuaged. Growers must spray weekly with strong mixtures. Many large commercial operations are planting as many as 100 pounds of seed per acre. Usually after 4 – 5 years the growing is complete. Upon which time the artificial shade is dismantled, the roots harvested, and new plots in new areas are prepared.

Shade

When building artificial shade you need only create a structure that shields ginseng plants from the top, or a roof-like cover breaking up the sunlight. The sides of the structure are kept open for air circulation. The goal is to dampen 70 – 80 percent of the sunlight. This is accomplished by cutting or obtaining boards that are about 2 inches wide that will be nailed to a wooden structure of 2 x 4s. In a way it is like laying down a hardwood floor but skipping every other board. After you have securely installed vertical beams (such as 4 x 4s) about every 10 feet around the gardens and attached a sturdy framework of 2 x 4s, you can attach the laths to the 2 x 4s for the roof. The space left between each lath should be about ¼ - ½ an inch before you attach the next parallel lath and so on. Some growers use snow fence because it almost has a ready-made lath characteristic. Make sure the lath-roof is about 6 – 8 feet from the plants (or higher if machinery has to access the crop).

Shade fabric such as polypropylene cloth can be purchased from some ginseng outfitters, which is even easier than wood to build shade out of, but it is expensive. Never use burlap because it will not allow the air to circulate or naturally cool the plants satisfactorily.

Drainage & Soil

Field cultivated ginseng in many ways is very artificial, since the grower creates the shade, and sometimes the soil, which establishes the drainage. When the soil of the plot is lacking, additional soil can be trucked in, disinfected of potential fungus, then mixed with leaf mold in raised beds with the existing field soil, and then any amendments are added as needed. If the soil of the potential plot is favorable in all respects except drainage then sand or small stones can be added to facilitate better drainage.

Disadvantages: The high start-up cost of supplies including building materials, chemicals, labor, machinery, and large amounts of seed are a disincentive. You need to harvest and dry a massive amount of root to break a profit, this requires far more work than required in woods-grown. The market value has been substantially diminished over the years for field cultivated ginseng. If 200 roots are required to make a dry pound (the range is 100 – 300 roots) at $20 a pound, then tens of thousands of roots are required to be harvested to make it a viable endeavor. Growers with diverse backgrounds of differing abilities and resources calculate a break-even amount needed per pound at auction to make it a logical choice. For instance a farmer with large machinery, extra land, a woodshop to build lath shade, and already purchasing chemicals in bulk, will find it easier to squeeze a profit as opposed to the novice grower considering field cultivation who has to rent land, buy machinery, and begin from scratch.

Also, diseases spread quickly due to the close proximity of the plants and the cost of constant spraying in both labor and supplies can be very high. If you live near a commercial operation, especially if you reside in or close to the state of Wisconsin, which currently is the largest commercial ginseng producing state, it would behoove you to visit a facility and get an idea of the demands it entails before you consider pursuing it.

CHAPTER III

Soil

The Preferred Range of pH for Ginseng 5.5 – 6.5
The Ideal pH Range 5.6 – 5.8

Needed supplies:
1) Soil Testing Kit
2) Soil Samples for Professional Testing

A) Working the Soil

Two of the three most important aspects of successful ginseng growing, **SDS** (**Shade**, **Drainage**, **Soil**), are related to the soil. These are its components of drainage and composition. A grower must be able to analyze what they have to work with in respect to soil pH and nutrients. Therefore as an important element in successful ginseng cultivation we must discuss soil. In this chapter we cover how to test it to ensure your crop will have the best chance at success and how to alter it if it needs to be changed or amended to meet the needs of growing and sustaining healthy ginseng plants.

(i) Analyzing the Soil
Before you create gardens and before acquiring rootlets or seed, you should first test the soil of the potential growing areas. Otherwise you may be without the land necessary to support anything but the expensive field cultivated style of growing. Ginseng demands that soil not only drain well but also have calcium, potassium, and phosphorus, along with a suitable pH. The good news is soil can be amended within reason. However if it must be done, you may need to amend it before you plant.

Otherwise phosphate you add will remain on the top layer and will not reach the roots where it is needed. Furthermore a grower should test before they plant because the most arduous step of ginseng cultivation is garden preparation and it would be folly beyond words to create that garden in poor soil. This chapter may give superfluous information to the experienced horticulturist nonetheless in an effort to prevent people from being blindsided we intend to be thorough.

By now you likely have an idea that ginseng prefers, a soil texture that is moist, well-drained, loose, rich, and loamy. Preferably a soil with generous amounts of leaf mold from decomposing wood, bark, leaves, and plants. Soil that when you handle it in your hands has a noticeably rich dark color. Also a soil that does not support standing water or contain too much clay, sand, and stones. Companion plants may help you hone in on an area where a patch may be viable however still inspect the potential plot for too much direct sun. If you are only dabbling with wild-simulated methods then depending on how much you want to invest in your experimentation, planting near companion plants while adhering to the 70 percent shade rule may suffice. Whatever your endeavor, we recommend at least purchasing a modest soil testing kit from a garden supply store to check the pH. They generally are easy to use and not too expensive ranging from $2 - $25 depending on the amount of extras you want with it and from where you purchase it. For about $15 if you shop around you can obtain the very simple to operate meter-kits that just require you to stab a probe into a sample of soil mixed with water. These are much quicker and easier to use than the less expensive dye-based kits.

The pH rating is a measure of the acidity or alkalinity in the soil. On this scale there is a range of $0 - 14$.

0 - 7 = Acidic (acidity increases as the number lowers)
- 7 - = Neutral
7 - 14 = Increasingly basic or alkaline

The Soil Test Kit

Whether you opt for a kit with a meter or traditional dye-testing, by following the instructions you should be able to get a sense of what you are working with. The pH will likely change from location to location so you will need to get several samples from an area slated for gardening, this makes the meter and probe easier to work with and it is generally more accurate. The range of 6.0 – 7.0 usually allows the best solubility of nutrients and preferred minerals. However ginseng likes the soil slightly more acidic preferring a 5.5 – 6.5 pH range. This is not too surprising when one considers that most of the nutrients and minerals in the soil can be absorbed into the root with the help of the extra acidity, which helps break them down more efficiently by making the nutrients soluble. Everything has its limits in nature and ginseng is no different. When ginseng plants are growing in soil that is too acidic they are under stress and more vulnerable to disease also their yield suffers, this begins when the pH drops below 5.5.

Professional Soil Analysis

If you have found that your soil is within the range for ginseng (5.5 – 6.5), then you may proceed with clearing the woods or planting however it is highly advisable that another step is completed for optimal results, a soil analysis. For a modest fee your local university or county extension of the Department of Agriculture should be able to perform this task. Usually it requires a small sample of soil, a completion of a form describing the crop you are planting, a fee ($10 - $20), and it is then sent by mail or dropped off at the testing center. After several weeks you will receive a detailed breakdown of what ginseng prefers and what your land supplying the sample offers. This step is extremely helpful to discover whether you need to add amendments.

The following table lists the ideal criteria that the soil-sample (for the crop of ginseng) will be measured against. Notice the

"target range" of the pH here is more liberal than the standard
preferred range of 5.5 – 6.5.

Components	Target Range
PH	5.15 – 6.66
Organic Matter	5.65
Nitrogen	112.0
Phosphorous	95.0
Potash	235.0
Calcium	1150.0
Magnesium	95.0
Sulfur	69.6
Sodium	35.0
Copper	.50
Iron	234.0
Manganese	4.50
Zinc	2.50
Boron	1.25
Aluminum	75.70
Molybdenum	3.20

(ii) Amending and Fertilizing Your Soil
This information obtained from the soil analysis is invaluable
when it is used to help decide what amendments to add in order
to create the best soil possible for ginseng and goldenseal.
Technically when discussing soil additives we should state
that a fertilizer is a treatment for the soil that has Nitrogen (N),
Phosphorous (P), and Potassium (K), as its constituents. This is
indicated on the label by percentage with the familiar number-
chain such as 15-15-15. In contrast a treatment for the soil that is
not composed of any Nitrogen, Phosphorous, or Potassium but
does contain important nutrients is classified as an amendment.
Lime is an example of a soil amendment. For simplicity and
clarity we use "amending" as a term of art in this manual. It is

far more important that the reader understand what to add than worry about its technical classification. Some of the most important amendments are:

Granulated Lime → Lowers the Acidity in the Soil
Phosphate → Helps Promote Plant Growth
Potash → Helps Promote the Plant's Immune System

Due to the infinite combinations that may be specifically relevant to your soil needs and the exact amount of what you decide to add, information on specific amounts is best deduced from the information supplied on respective labels and charts at garden stores for each product accordingly. However since lime, phosphate, and potash are common amendments they are covered in more detail.

Granulated Lime offers many attributes. If your plots are below 5.0 on the pH scale then add lime before planting and in later years as needed after the growing season. It is added to raise the pH or lower the acidity in your potential garden plot. Accompanying lime amending-treatment comes calcium, magnesium, and an increased pace of decay of organic matter, which is advantageous adding nitrogen to the soil.

When amending with lime, if you are eager to raise the pH by .5, then for every square yard amend with 4-ounces of hydrated lime on average soils. It may not be wise to try to amend your soil if you are in the lower 6 range of the pH scale since 5.6 – 5.8 is what ginseng ideally prefers.

Potash does not offer calcium like lime does but it can be used to reduce the acidity of the soil. An excellent source of potash is found in ashes from wood, and like lime, they can be applied during garden preparation or at the end of the growing season.

Seasonal broadcasting of wood ash (for instance collected from a furnace that burns firewood) is an excellent way of applying potash. It is easy enough to apply by simply broadcasting a light coating preferably by hand on a dry and still day. Do not do this when the plants have emerged unless you are careful not to get the ash stuck on the plant leaflets. Another advantage of the wood ash is that it seems to discourage slug activity.

If calcium levels are still lagging then Bone Meal can be added. It offers a great source of calcium. Calcium nitrate is another suitable amendment. The importance of calcium cannot be understated even with the soil pH far above and below the 5.5 – 6.5 range, healthy roots in the extremes are found to possess higher levels of calcium. Calcium has also been linked to producing roots that are more robust.

If the Soil is Too Sweet

Generally, prior to planting, if the soil needs to be amended it is to decrease the acidity but if the soil is too sweet then acquirer an acidifying agent like aluminum sulfate.

(iii) Amending After the Garden has been Planted

From observation and knowledge of the soil ratings in the gardens there may be a time when you feel the plants are in need of help through soil amending. Some overt signs may be stunted growth or a plant that is more pea green than the normal healthy greenish hue. Fortunately this can be remedied.

While the application of wood ash can become a regular task despite any appearance of plant deficiencies, the other amending is done when there seems to be deficiencies in established gardens. If the plants look malnourished or from the initial soil tests the numbers were borderline, you can add hydrated lime to raise a pH that is too low. Additionally Miracle-Gro as a foliar fertilizer is an excellent source of food for established plants. Using the 15-30-15 rating add 1-tablespoon per 1-gallon of water (or 1-tablespoon to each 1-gallon of mix if it is being added to a mixture of fungicide) into your sprayer and apply once a month during the growing season.

It is also wise to subsequently test the soil of the gardens especially if the plant quality is consistently lacking. If the soil is depleted of phosphorus there is the alternative of triple superphosphate that can be carried down to the roots with the rain. Try the 0-40-0 rated formula and refer to the package to establish the amount needed to apply.

(iv) Fertilizing Established Gardens

Avoid the application of garden fertilizer to the surface of the garden after the seeds have been planted. Indeed the potash component is good however the phosphate will stay on the topsoil instead of reaching the roots (unless the phosphate applied is triple superphosphate). Therefore with conventional garden fertilizer the nitrogen filters down facilitating greater growth mainly in the plant top, which is not ideal.

All fertilizer should be used miserly if you are trying to practice woods-grown or wild-simulated otherwise you will end up with at best a root that more resembles a much lesser valued field cultivated or at worst produce a plant that is vulnerable to disease for having grown too fast. Some growers will apply a 1-tablespoon to 1-gallon water mixture of Miracle-Gro several times during the summer. We will do this if a particular patch despite having the proper shade and moisture appears malnourished. The key for valuable non-field cultivated ginseng is slow and healthy root growth. Never fertilize with animal dung. Furthermore avoid livestock manure because it is full of seeds, disease, and can reputedly augment the flavor of the root.

CHAPTER IV

Creating Gardens

Suggested Attributes of the Site:
1) Shade: 70% from a Hardwood Canopy
2) Soil: Rich & Loamy with Good Drainage
3) pH range: 5.5 – 6.5

After investing the necessary mental energy to plan where the best potential gardens should be, by carrying out the preliminary testing on the soil, analyzing the shade, and being satisfied by the drainage, it is time to put your planning into action. Ginseng may prefer a northeastern slope, certainly an eastern facing slope is ideal however if your land faces the west or south just make sure that the shade and drainage are adequate.

Beginning to create the gardens in the early part of summer or late spring is advisable because it offers plenty of time to prepare for the fall planting season. If you tackle this project for spring planting be sure it is completed before May begins and if in the fall make sure the operation is completed prior to the ground freezing for the year. The creation of gardens can be very strenuous depending on the land that is chosen to work with, be sure you and your workers are physically fit for the task. There is no eloquent manner to discuss and describe this part of the operation. In this chapter we cover the construction of the gardens, the planting of the seed or rootlets, mulching, and upkeep.

You should have the following to complete this step:
1) Rototiller – preferably rear tined and at least 4 ½ horsepower
2) Chainsaw

3) Brush pruners
4) Hard rake
5) Single pointed hard-soil hoe also called a Warren hoe
6) Stratified seed or rootlets
7) Fungicide: Manzate 200 (or bleach)
8) Water for disinfecting seeds and a rinsing solution
9) Fertilizer
10) Mulch: sawdust, straw, shredded leaves
11) Slug poison

A) Getting Started and Breaking Ground

First armed with a chainsaw and brush pruners begin by clearing unnecessary segments of the underbrush this includes shrubs, dead trees, saplings, any trees you do not need for shade, as well as low branches that will impede air circulation and prove annoying. When removing the lower branches do not allow any remaining to be lower than 7 - 8 feet, again unless they are necessary for providing shade. This plot should be under hardwoods, thus remove any pine trees that are not absolutely necessary for shade. Pine needles will continue to descend and sour the soil if the tree remains. Make sure any areas with accumulated pine needles are not too sour by testing the pH levels.

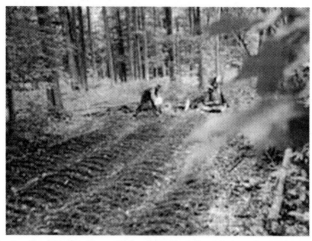

Garden Construction: Rows Being Scratched, Seed Being Planted (above)

Garden Construction: Sawdust Applied as Final Step,
Notice Garden Layout Changes Depending on Natural Conditions
(Trees/Shade, Rocks, Slope, etc) (below)

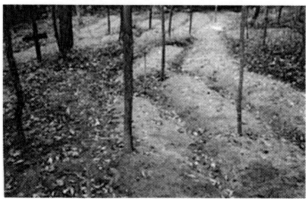

After clearing the brush and any unnecessary larger trees it is time to remove any weeds and smaller plants. Although herbicides may make this step easier, they may not be legal in your state or province. Also customers prefer ginseng as chemical-free as possible. A rototiller in our estimation is an absolute must for medium to large cultivation. If possible buy, borrow, rent, or obtain a rear-tine rototiller. This machine will pull the weeds, rocks, and small tree trunks in the manner needed for the operation.

Although a rototiller is advisable, if you are only planting a pound or less, or the land is not conducive to operating a rototiller, then traditional implements can be used but it will be substantially more labor intensive to work the ground. Note that after your gardens are tilled and trenched, the tiller will not be needed until the creation of more gardens therefore it may be feasible to rent one.

When using a rototiller try to cultivate on land where it can be safely operated. We have operated ours on some fairly steep slopes but one must always employ common sense. Ginseng likes steep hillsides in the wild, but you will be creating a garden that needs to be cared for and worked with, so be reasonable. If the land chosen offers great hardwoods but no appreciable grade then increased drainage will be achieved by creating domes and raised beds, which will be discussed in this chapter.

To safely and efficiently operate the tiller, run it up and down the slope of the hill also keep a firm grip on the handles which will likely buck and jump when the tines come into contact with stones and roots. Try to reach a depth of about 6 - 8 inches. The soil should be broken up to a satisfactory level after the third time the tiller covers the plot but this depends on your soil. The tilling can be done in one day if the garden is being prepared in late August shortly before planting, or you can pace yourself in intervals throughout the summer. Generally by the third tilling the soil should be loose like that of a vegetable garden although it depends on the site since some people may have to till more to get the desired loose-soil consistency. Make sure to remove as many of the rocks (larger than a baseball) that get kicked up as possible and till as close to the hardwood trees as their respective roots will allow. Obviously you do not want to damage important roots of your shade trees. The roots of these trees will eventually work into the gardens, that fact has to be accepted. You need their shade and their roots will continue to grow over time. Also smaller rocks and stones can remain because they can help with drainage. However if the potential garden is composed of mostly rock the site may need to be abandoned unless large amounts of loamy soil are brought in to get the balance of at least 65 percent rich soil to 35 percent rock.

If all conditions are good but the soil consistency is less than satisfactory try tilling in large amounts of organic matter (e.g. shredded leaves, bark, naturally decayed wood) early in the summer so that it has time to decay. A layer of two inches of shredded leaves tilled into the potential garden is an ideal enrichment if the soil is slightly lacking. Before the final tilling which is best just prior to the planting of the seed (within a couple of days), you will want to add any soil amendments if they are needed. The touchstone for this will be determined by the soil testing remembering that a pH of 5.6 - 5.8 is the best and the range of 5.5 – 6.5 is acceptable. If your soil tests low for phosphorus add superphosphate 0-20-0 or Bone Meal (for every 100 square feet of garden add 1-pound of superphosphate or 2-pounds of Bone Meal). Do this before tilling because superphosphate will not be taken down with rainwater so you have to place it into the soil where the roots will be, unlike nitrogen, triple superphosphate and potash, which will seep down with rainwater. Also when adding soil amendments, always amend the whole area cleared.

Even if the tilling is efficiently finished early in the summer, you will have to go back and till the site shortly before planting, which will break the soil up and eradicate any weeds that began growing during the interim. So just assume that the final till will be in late August or early September and that will be the time to add any amendments or any further decomposed leaf mold if it is needed. Never add oak leaves or pine needles because they can sour your soil for the most part leaf mold is one of the best natural additives to enrich the soil.

B) Constructing the Actual Garden

The most arduous part has been completed. Now that the clearing, tilling, and amendments, have been tended to, it is the time to analyze the plot and decide how you want the actual gardens to run. Much like an artist, this is your canvas, you only need to comport to the basic rules on drainage and size. The gardens must run up and down the slop of the land for the best drainage. Aim for gardens of about four feet in width and the length can be however far is prudent. At this stage, you have some degree of discretion and freedom to work with your environment. Four feet is a practical width because you can spray, weed, kneel-over, and remove diseased plants or debris with ease. But to utilize all available space sometimes a garden may bulge an extra foot or two in various places. The garden length and width is sometimes predicated on the plot especially by stubborn tree stumps, trunks comprising the canopy, and large boulders that are just not worth moving. Work with the environment but definitely try not to let the gardens generally be wider than the four feet mark.

(i) Spacing and Trenching of Gardens
Spacing
   After the clearing has been completed try to keep the gardens separated by about 12 – 18 inches from one garden to the next. You want to be able to utilize this swath as a pathway without it being awkward therefore if you are not sure-footed perhaps extend it to two feet, remember once these gardens are planted you do not want to have to step inside them. If plenty of space has been cleared under the forest canopy and you are planning a large-scale operation then the pathways can be widened to a suitable size to allow for machinery to be driven between gardens especially for spraying. However for most small to medium size growers this will not be necessary.

Trenching

The last use of the rototiller on the garden site is to dig a trench on the border of the tracks that will be the actual gardens. With a cultivator mounted on the back of the tiller (it looks like a v-plow) you will make trenches up and down the slope of the plot on the outside border of the planned gardens. Again work with the land not against it, for example stop the garden and trench at a large tree trunk if it is in the middle of the garden track. Then begin a new garden and trench making the tree merely an island in that garden. Continue making the trenches, which will be the actual exterior borders of the gardens. Depending on the soil, you may have to run the tiller several times up the trench to obtain the 6 – 8 inches desired for the width and 6 – 8 inches of depth needed for it. These will create a perfect vector for the runoff of excess water away from the plants.

Additionally while the tiller is still handy, start at the highest point of the land that has been cleared and create diversion trenches that will guide water away from the gardens altogether. This in an effort to facilitate the drainage of excess water from heavy storms or spring runoff, it may sound paranoid but ginseng does not tolerate wet conditions while potentially devastating fungi revel in it.

C) Making the Rows

By this point in the procedure, the cleared forest plots should have been tilled at least three times, garden-borders trenched, and it should be within days of actual planting. After placing the finishing touches or doming on the plot, like a vegetable garden, create some rows for the seeds. By far this is one of the more enjoyable aspects of planting.

(i) Raised Beds and Doming the Garden

It is now time for "doming" the garden. With a hard-rack in hand, pull the extra soil brought up by the trenching tool or cultivator, that is already present from making the exterior trenches, towards the middle of the garden beds. By tapering the soil into the garden it creates a dome shape. If you do not have any significant grade now is the time to create raised beds. First it is advisable on flat terrain to add mulch to the soil to aid with drainage. Early in the summer, preceding the fall planting, dump a two-inch layer of finely shredded hardwood leaf mulch if possible over the site and till it into the area to help create a very loose soil. While still adhering to the four feet width rule, the length as with regular gardens, can be tailored to convenience. On the outside create a deeper than usual trench and this soil will be incorporated into the garden, raising it above ground level. With raised beds, the exterior trench should be about a foot wide and have a depth of about eight inches. This should provide enough extra soil to establish a modest but necessary grade.

One more obscure planting method that may work for smaller amounts of seed on flat grades is to make small mounds. After completing the garden, every foot, work the soil into a 5 – 7 inch diameter mound and plant four seeds in the mound. We still however prefer the raised bed method when there is not a preexisting slop to work with.

(ii) Scratching Rows
Quick Reference for (ii) Scratching Rows and (iii) Planting Seed
Garden Spacing: 1 Seed Every 4 - 5 Inches in Rows 6 - 10 Inches Apart
Seedbed Spacing: 1 Seed Every 1 - 1½ Inches in Rows 6 - 8 Inches Apart
Transplanting Rootlets: 1 Rootlet Every 6 - 8 Inches in Rows 8 - 10 Inches Apart

The decision on the distance between rows as well as spacing between seed in the rows is based on your goals. Early on when we began planting ginseng the only reference available were articles from outdoors magazines on ginseng growing, within the past twenty years several excellent books and numerous sites on the Internet now offer their rules of spacing. Much of them are the same, they suggest a range of inches of what is considered acceptable. Of course it is easy to get lured into the idea of being able to plant 100 pounds of seed (estimate 7,000 seeds per pound) in an acre of garden space, if only the seeds are planted about one inch apart in line-rows that are six inches from each other. Then after two years of growing they are then transplanted to permanent gardens and you are only 3 - 4 years from a colossal fortune. Do not be fooled by this. If growing ginseng were as easy as growing onions it would not demand the price that it does on the world market.

Stratified seed will likely have a germination rate ranging between 70 - 90 percent and in theory transplanting rootlets to permanent gardens after the attrition of nature has thinned them out (usually after their second growing season) makes perfect sense. However given the atrocious record we have had with transplanting healthy roots only to have them do poorly in their new permanent gardens, we only transplant for emergencies. If you have the space, we strongly endorse planting your seed with permanent spacing from the outset.

That being said it is time to do your spacing. After doming is completed, take the hard-soil hoe and begin scratching rows. Again the garden should run down the slop of the land, like the nose on a human face, but the rows inside the garden will run perpendicular with the outside long-trenches, like the mouth on the human face. Create rows every 6 - 8 inches, if space is unlimited then a row every 8 - 10 inches is better. The larger spacing will make it more difficult when disease strikes for it to spread. Root rot alone requires the removal of plants at least 18 inches from infected plants in every direction, even if they appear to be healthy. However larger spacing does mean more resources are needed to create and maintain the garden. A pound of seeds (which remember can range between 6,500 – 8,500 seeds) can chew up a lot of property if you plant it too sparse. It is unlikely that every seed will yield a plant, which is why so many growers prefer planting the seeds into a seedbed for the first year or two. However the scale and style of planting depends on your decision. It never hurts to experiment by planting some seeds in temporary seedbeds and leaving others planted in permanent gardens upon initial sowing.

Once you have finished scratching all the rows, before the seed is placed in them, take 15-15-15 plant fertilizer and superphosphate 0-20-0 (this is the second superphosphate application since you likely would have added some during the final rototilling) combine the two together in a mixture whereby 50 percent of the mixture is plant fertilizer and 50 percent is superphosphate. Then sprinkle sparingly the fertilizer mix in each newly created row. This step may be omitted for those attempting to grow an organic crop or if one is satisfied with the level of existing nutrients present in the soil.

(iii) Planting Seed

Assuming you have disinfected the seeds (e.g. 1-tablespoon Manzate to 1-gallon water, *see* Chapter V Seed) it is time to commence seeding the gardens. Place the seed in the rows with one seed every 4 - 5 inches. This will result in a good concentration. If the decision is to plant a dense seedbed for yearlings with the intent to transplant the roots at a later date, then plant a seed every 1 – 1½ inch. Make sure the soil that you are placing the seed into is not too dry. It should be dark brown and moist. If experiencing a dry spell while you are forced to plant, then dump a small amount of water in the rows before the seed is placed into the ground and promptly cover the seed with soil. Avoid having the outer case of the seed dry-out because it can prevent germination in the spring.

Next after your seeds have been placed in the rows, standing in between the gardens with a hard-rake in hand, begin to cover them. Use the topside of the rake that features the long smooth edge (not the teeth-side) and begin working it across the row, reaching over and with a series of 45-degree angle strokes, carefully covering the seeds with about ¾ - 1 inch of soil. After covering the seeds, gently tamp the soil down to help the dirt fill in around the seeds and flush out any existing pockets of air that may dry them out. This is easily done by holding the rake handle in a vertical position and applying the end of the rake against the soil in a downward motion.

D) Mulching

After the seeds are sown and covered with soil, it is time to place some insulation over the gardens to replicate nature with its leaves. Applying mulch is the best way to help the plants and surrounding soil maintain optimal moisture levels and temperatures during the extremes reached in both winter and summer. The preferred soil temperature during the growing season should be in the middle 60s (Fahrenheit). Mulch helps moderate the summer heat and encourages the ground to withhold moisture and prevent it from becoming too dry while also deterring weeds, and absorbing the force of heavy downpours. Furthermore by absorbing the pounding of rain showers mulch can help prevent fungi from being splashed on nearby plants. Most growers use dry leaves, sawdust, and straw. A combination of dry shredded leaves and a hardwood sawdust cover is the best formula.

(i) Shredded Leaves

Applying a blanket of chopped hardwood leaves is the best mulch. This is where it helps to plan ahead because chances are you will be planting before the leaves fall. Therefore if some leaves shredded and bagged from the prior year are present it makes things much easier. Shredded leaves are better than whole leaves because when dry the bigger leaves are easily removed by wind and when drenched they pose a problem for fragile yearlings trying to grow through their blanket-like cover during the following spring. Also shredded leaves readily breakdown and enrich the soil.

(ii) Straw

If you are without a supply of dry leaves, chopped straw will work. Utilize oat straw instead of wheat. This is because invariably some oat and wheat seeds will be among the straw and one does not want this growing in with the ginseng. The oat seed will not survive the winter but the wheat seed is capable of remaining viable. Therefore oat straw is best. Nonetheless leaves are by far better and should remain the first choice. So if you can procure dry, shredded hardwood leaves, just not too much oak because of its souring tendency, it will be more advantageous. Use straw with caution, it seems that straw makes a more hospitable habitat for slugs and snails.

(iii) Application of Mulch
Mulch on Stratified Seed

The application of mulch changes to meet the needs of the garden. First, when planting stratified seed you do not want more than ½ inch of mulch present and covering the seeds

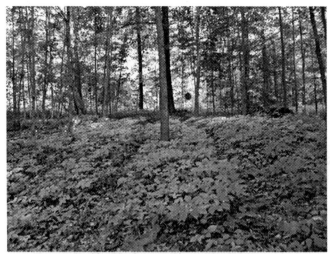

Healthy Woodsgrown Ginseng Garden &
Environment Modified to Ideal Balance (above)

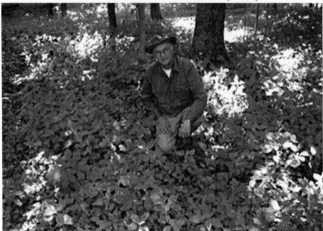

Ginseng Plants Eventhough Sparsely Planted Can Appear Dense (above)

before the spring growth. If your winters are fairly mild, then you need only apply ½ - ¾ of an inch of mulch in the fall. If your winters are more severe then about a 1½ inch application works well. As long as you rake off the excess in early spring so that by early May the yearlings will be able to pierce through the ground and through the ½ inch of remaining mulch. Once they have, then as needed go back on a dry day and add more mulch around the plants where you think it is lacking. For instance if one area is drying out at a faster pace than other parts of the garden, then apply an extra ¼ inch. Do this on a dry day to prevent the new mulch from adhering to the leaves of the plants.

Mulch on Rootlets or Mature Plants

If you are planting rootlets then you should apply 1½ - 2 inches of mulch for the winter, while allowing ¾ - 1 inch to remain during the growing season beginning in early May. Mature plants are stronger and will be able to grow through straw and shredded leaves. Again by the spring before the growing season inspect the beds and make sure that whatever has been applied has not matted down too thick. Again this is why large unshredded leaves should be avoided because they adhere together like wet newspapers by springtime creating an almost impossible layer to penetrate through, especially for goldenseal seedlings and ginseng yearlings.

(iv) Sawdust

After finishing the application of leaves or straw, hardwood sawdust is a desired final layer. Usually this can be procured from a local sawmill. Apply a coarse style of sawdust preferably since smooth sawdust tends to mat and the coarse dust helps deter slugs (a major enemy). Covering the garden with a very thin layer over the leaves or straw will suffice. In fact 20, 5-gallon buckets of sawdust covers about 130 x 4 feet of garden (if ordering the sawdust from a sawmill that is about "2.2 yards" of sawdust). The sawdust layer also helps prevent the wind from removing the leaf mulch that has been applied. As mentioned, since sawdust has a tendency to mat if it is used to too heavy, it really should be used as complementary mulch along with leaves or straw and always as just a light covering.

E) Final Steps

Next broadcast some slug pellets on top of the final mulch layer. Then for gardens made in the fall, forge for some bushy-full branches that may have been trimmed off the nearby trees. Choose branches that are easy enough to handle and devoid of leaves making sure they are long enough to sit onto the new gardens over the sawdust. These will be removed in the spring prior to the growing season when you inspect the gardens and mulch. They help provide a bit of a weight on the mulch against wind gusts and even act as a temporary snow fence. Snow during the winter is your friend because it is a natural insulator protecting the roots from extreme cold. Furthermore these bushy branches also help against deer walking through your gardens.

Congratulations, you are done until the spring. Creating gardens can easily be the most physically enervating of the steps in growing ginseng and planting thousands of seeds may even border on the tedious side, however if you pace yourself and chip away little by little it can be very rewarding. We feel under the right circumstances time spent laboring in the woods is far superior to time squandered sitting in traffic and some even derive a strength from working with the soil.

Anyway remember by spring much of the mulch will be raked off, since after the winter you only want the ground to be covered about one inch for reemerging roots and ½ an inch for yearlings. Especially if fall planting occurred before the leaves from the natural canopy had yet to descend.

Grower's Tip!

Here is some parting advice with mulch. First, we do not recommend using straw. Many growers use it and seem to like it however it harbors slugs, and they will be one of your most indefatigable enemies. Secondly, like other things with ginseng, the mulch may not be as crucial as we believe. We get cold winters and occasionally there are places in the gardens during the spring that were scraped bare of their mulch over the winter. Promptly an inch of shredded leaves is applied shortly before the plants began to reemerge to prevent the area from becoming too warm and dry. Still without this mulch-aegis for the winter the plants often survive. The point is that although one should take every precaution to limit risks preventing a successful crop, this plant will surprise you with its vitality as well as with its weakness.

There will likely be places that everything was done right but nothing grew for a host of unknown reasons and unanswered explanations. Many years back we planted a seemingly perfect garden in the fall that did not yield a single plant by the following spring, disgusted beyond words with our piteous results we left the plot to nature instead of tilling it up and trying again. The next year we noticed a vast crop of yearlings emerging from this previously assumed dead plot. We had been sold green instead of stratified seed, were too inexperienced then to notice the difference, and unwittingly planted it.

On one occasion we had gardens that only produced an extremely small percentage of ginseng of what was planted, that fall they were rototilled up and made into goldenseal plots. The following growing season a surprising amount of ginseng survived the rototilling and replanting of the area, happily coexisting among the new goldenseal that grew. Later testing showed that despite being adjacent to excellent garden space the garden that gave the terrible ginseng was obscenely low in phosphorous. Therefore do not be afraid to do several soil tests of a large area.

F) Seedbeds and Transplanted Roots

Quick Reference and Review
Seedbed Spacing: 1 Seed Every 1 – 1½ Inches in Rows 6 – 8
Inches Apart
Transplanted Roots: 1 Rootlet Every 6 – 8 Inches in Rows 8
– 10 Inches Apart

As noted earlier if you are inclined to plant a seedbed first, then later transplant the roots after the first or second growing season, in some ways it can be advantageous. When ginseng plants are growing in a seedbed it clearly is easier maintaining and spraying the crop. However, again, we strongly advise against this method to those just starting out, having ourselves lost over 14,000 healthy two-year old rootlets when we were novice growers transplanting them. Transplanting does not always proceed as smooth as other publications like to portray. We followed all the recommendations but still lost most of that section of our crop and with ginseng it takes years to recover. If you are intrepid or are cramped on space and choose this method then employ the physical paradigm of creating gardens discussed hitherto for creating seedbeds, but plant more dense. A seed every 1 – 1½ inch within the rows, and rows 6 - 8 inches apart is good for seedbeds.

If transplanting roots then make sure the bud of the root is not damaged in transit and facing towards the surface when it is placed in the row for planting. Also while the roots are in transit keep them moist with damp (but not soaking wet) cloth to prevent them from drying-out, old towels work well to this end. The root may be set horizontal before being covered with the soil although we prefer to plant the roots vertical thereby showing no evidence of them being transplanted. The vertical root will more resemble a wild one, which is more desirable and marketable. Exercise care during transplantation of roots, do it while they are dormant after the plant tops have wilted and turned yellow. Like when planting seeds this operation should be carried out either in the fall or early spring, unless you have to perform emergency transplanting on a diseased or damaged plant during the summer.

The rows will be dug deeper to accommodate the longer root. Instead of scratched rows being 1 – ¾ of an inch deep for seeds, you will have to merely create deeper rows, which should not be more difficult because the soil will be loose from proper rototilling. It is basic math, if two-year old roots are three inches long then scratch rows that are four inches deep to accommodate the root and allow the inch of soil to cover it.

Space the roots about 6 - 8 inches apart in the rows and keep the rows about 8 –10 inches apart. If garden space is an issue then six inches can separate the rows. It is all a gamble because in theory the roots, assuming they were handled correctly during transplanting and the conditions of the new gardens are ideal, should have a great success rate. Sparse planting helps deter disease while dense planting is easier maintenance unless disease strikes. Experiment and find what works best for you while weighing the risks. However if you have the resources always avoid dense planting.

G) Quarantine Beds

When creating main gardens it is a good idea to have some small ones located in an isolated area of your woods for plants that may develop disease later on. Invariably disease will strike your crop, while prevention is the goal, containment is the solution after it hits. For example there are times when you want to remove a plant from a garden to prevent the spread of disease however the root of the afflicted plant may survive and come up healthy next year. Without a quarantine bed your only choice is to extract the plant and hastily place the root in unfavorable conditions or let the root die outright, but with a place to plant it, you give the ginseng a chance to grow again. However this quarantine bed must be below, far enough away, and not upwind, of the healthy gardens or you may end up tripping over dollars to pick up pennies if you risk disease spreading into the healthy ginseng populations. Obviously these gardens can greatly deviate from the standard garden size and be placed in areas that otherwise did not offer enough space for a full garden.

H) General Upkeep

It is wise to inspect your gardens if you can get to them at regular intervals during the winter especially if there is unseasonably warm weather. The roots and seeds will remain safe if properly planted and mulched under normal winter conditions. But take note of excessive warming and cooling just before or after the dead of winter or freak heavy rains which can actually bring on a fungi attack even outside of the growing season. You cannot control the weather but you can inspect your beds and add trenches (with a pick or shovel) or extra mulch if it is removed by wind or animals. Also be ready to clear debris from the drainage trenches if off-season rains bring substantial water.

(i) Healthy Habits

During the growing season you will be watching for disease and spraying a woods-grown crop every 10 – 14 days (or promptly after a heavy rainstorm). Observing plants that are getting too much sun, water, or displaying the reddish/yellow colors of disease will become part of your routine. Checking on mole activity, picking up branches that fall onto your gardens, and inspecting the mulch are also important tasks. As well as keeping an eye on the natural canopy making sure holes have not developed allowing too much sustained direct sunlight to filter in hitting the gardens. This may sound like a lot of information to keep track of but this upkeep will become second nature by the end of your first growing season.

(ii) Weeding

Finally weeding is another consideration. Weeds compete for water and nutrients. They can harbor and be a starting point for disease especially if they reduce proper airflow. Warm humid pockets of air near the ginseng are conditions that growers want to avoid. However they can also serve a vital role in a certain circumstance. Granted weeds are in direct competition in the gardens for moisture and soil nutrients with the ginseng. Thus during a drought and normal weather conditions they should be removed, but during excessive rainfall they serve a purpose. For instance if a summer is too wet, the weeds can absorb some of the extra water naturally out of the beds and they are cannon fodder for bugs especially slugs. Also if during the summer season a weather system sets up that keeps bringing rain and humid conditions you will need to spray heavy and often because fungi will be thriving. Removing weeds that are nevertheless helping to extract excess water from a wet garden may also broadcast spores previously embedded, thereby pulling them out of the soil and mulch allowing the spores to spread like a virtual Pandora's box. Usually weeds can be removed but if the summer gets unseasonably wet, then weigh the risks.

Chapter V

Ginseng Seed

Now that you are versed on how and where to plant ginseng the next step is to consider the manner in which you begin. Your options are to purchase either seed or rootlets. When buying seed from a ginseng dealer you are confronted with the option of buying seed at two different stages in development, stratified seed and green seed (or non-stratified seed). When purchasing rootlets you can purchase plants in either their second, third, and some cases even fourth growing season. Notwithstanding these options, which are explained in this chapter, the most logical beginning is with stratified seed.

From harvesting, stratifying, disinfecting, storing, and purchasing, this chapter will provide guidance on the important information every grower needs to know about seed.

A) Seed: Green Seed verses Stratified Seed

In Chapter I, when discussing the life cycle of the ginseng plant, we explained that the ginseng berry becomes ripe and drops from a mature plant in the late summer or early fall. Assuming this seed undergoes the necessary conditions precedent of warming and cooling to reach germination, the seed will not be ready to send a plant (or yearling) to the surface until about 19 - 21 months after it fell from the parent plant.

(i) Green Seed

When the ripened ginseng berry is removed from the plant the seeds inside are referred to as green seed. That means if you purchase green seed, which is usually about half the price of stratified seed when purchased by the pound, you will have to stratify it yourself or plant it green and wait an extra year for it to grow.

Unless one has an excess of time and land, planting green seed in gardens or seedbeds is highly inefficient. First your germination rate even with stratified seed ready to grow will likely only be 90 percent (assuming they were float tested) at best. With green seed you are not just fighting the variable of a seed developing properly but also it being consumed by the many enemies that dig, dwell, and live in the soil. Furthermore the construction of a garden and upkeep in regards to weed control, pest control, and spraying can be laborious. Therefore toiling an extra year without any plants to show for the work with seeds that though planted properly, may or may not produce a plant is difficult to justify.

Some growers buy green seed along with stratified seed in the fall. They then stratify the green separately while having the stratified seed to promptly plant in seedbeds. This system works well if you have good organizational skills and the time to execute it. We did this in the beginning and there is an advantage of knowing that even if there is a run on stratified seeds from the seed vendors you will have what you need ready to plant after the seed is ready.

Tricking Nature
There is a method to hasten germination of green seed that has been perfected by some enterprising and impressive ginseng experts most notably Robert Beyfuss of the Cornell Cooperative Extension (New York, USA) and John Proctor from the University of Guelph in Ontario, Canada. The trick is to turn green seed into viable seed in one winter. We have never dabbled in this project and thus cannot attest to its efficacy and given the amount invested in planting and preparation we suggest just purchasing stratified seed to the average grower since the savings is minimal. Nonetheless for academic reasons it is indeed worthy of mention.

Begin by harvesting and de-pulping seed upon its turning red in the late summer. Then disinfect (with 1-tablespoon Manzate 200 or bleach to 1-gallon water) and store the green seed in a moist sand mixture (like a stratification box) at a constant temperature of 60 degrees (Fahrenheit) until the very end of December. Next put your moist sand/seed mixture into a place where the temperature will remain at a constant 40 degrees (Fahrenheit) until late March or early April then plant the seed. By June, plants should emerge with reported germination rates of 40 – 50 percent. This is up to you, the grower, and how much you want to experiment with and invest into the project, but by all means for the novice stick to obtaining stratified seed.

(ii) Stratified Seed

Stratified seed is seed that has been through the first year of waiting. You purchase it in the fall for fall planting, and after hard work, proper sowing, and luck, the vast majority will germinate and send up a plant the following spring.

Stratified seed, like green seed, is usually best if purchased by the pound. Unless you are just dabbling and are planting a half or quarter pound of wild-simulated, it is wise to avoid purchasing seed in small amounts from a commercial nursery as the markup is usually obscene. Ideally if you are doing this as a hobby and hoping for reasonable financial returns then you want to do the maximum. That is to prepare, plant, and harvest as much as time, available resources, and nature allows you to accomplish. This is why planning is a key element to successful cultivation of ginseng. Whether you are going with artificial shade or utilizing the forest canopy, you must map out in your logbook how much garden or seedbed space is available because once you buy stratified seed it needs to be properly planted that fall or carefully stored and sown in the narrow window before May during the following spring.

Calculating How Much is Needed

With this estimation of available planting spots you can calculate your order. Usually seeds are sold by the pound but the actual amount of product received can vary substantially. Some pounds contain almost 8,500 seed while others only 6,500. This is due to seed size, one example is Northern seed tends to be slightly thicker than their Southern counterpart.

Therefore do some computations based on your plan. Assuming that you plant seedbeds first, then later transplant the surviving plants to gardens after their first or second growing year, then how much garden space is needed or even available? In an average pound of 7,500 seeds, planted in seedbeds four feet wide, rows every six inches, and a seed every inch in the row, work the math and you can start to get an idea of the space needed to be available for planting.

If you plant permanent gardens at the outset, which we strongly recommend, then you will be planting less dense and perhaps at least thrice as much space will be required per pound. Remember earlier that in permanent gardens your plot is generally four feet wide, with rows 6 – 10 inches apart (6 – 8 being normal and 8 – 10 ideal), and a seed every 4 - 5 inches in the rows. A good estimation of what is needed is a must, as you would not want to waste seed.

The Best Places to Purchase Seed

It is ideal to purchase seed from commercial sellers that are in your relative climate, although in theory Southern seed should grow fine in the North, winters in the northern United States and southern Canada can offer very cold temperatures however adequate mulching should provide more than enough protection. Northern seed generally has slightly more bulk to it, although again the right application of mulch to your planting site should, in theory, augment the cold as a factor. The Internet is an excellent resource for locating sellers and making price comparisons although sometimes the less commercial the vender is, the better their prices are. There are some seed sellers listed in the appendix if you do not have access to the Internet. Furthermore it is always wise to shop around because prices fluctuate among the vendors as supplies and inventories change from year to year.

B) Care for Purchased Seed

In the beginning curiosity demanded that when the seed arrived we would always measure it with simple measuring implements used for cooking. From teaspoon, to tablespoon, to cup, this helped us evaluate how many seeds we had to work with.

On Average:
1-Teaspoon = 60 seeds
1-Tablespoon = 180 seeds
1-Coffee container labeled 13 ounces will hold 10,000 seeds; three 13-ounce coffee cans hold four pounds of seed

Upon receiving your seed either in the mail or after returning home from acquiring them in person you must prevent them from drying out. It is likely that your gardens are just about complete but your seeds need to be stored a couple of days while you execute the final touches. Therefore divide and inspect the seeds in a manner that does not allow them to dehydrate.

This can be accomplished by taking a 1-cup cooking measurer and begin dividing the seeds by placing them into Ziploc bags (or similarly styled plastic bags). The seeds should look light brownish or tan and be firm. If it is slightly split with fine root fibers pushing out from the core it is okay. Seeds that are mushy and soft should be immediately discarded. While it is not expected that one or several buyers can evaluate 7,000 – 60,000 seeds in a quick period, an optical frisk will usually suffice. The objective of the inspection is to make sure an unacceptable percentage of seeds are not spoiled upon arrival.

After inspection and division into the 1-cup servings place the seed into the refrigerator. Keep the bags zipped to prevent seed dehydration, however if they are in refrigeration more than two days take them out, unzip the bag, and for a few minutes move the seeds around with your hand (make sure your hands are clean). Then seal them up and place the bags back into the refrigerator. The day the seeds are planted you will perform a step to disinfect them by mixing the seed with a 1-tablespoon Manzate 200 to 1-gallon of water mixture or the less favorable 1-tablespoon bleach to 1-gallon water mix (explained later in this chapter). Given the condition of tens of thousands of seeds held in moist sandy-soil to be sold by commercial ginseng sellers to perspective buyers like yourself it is very wise to kill any disease, especially fungi, that may be traveling on your seeds before planting them.

C) Seed Harvested From Mature Plants

At some point in this endeavor you will likely acquire some ginseng berries either early on from a grower helping you out or from your own plants in substantial numbers when they reach their third and fourth growing season. A few plants may even produce seed in their second season depending on the root size of the respective plant, but usually it is the mature plants that yield significant fruits. Given that 3 – 4 year old plants send up seed clusters of 30 berries or more, with 1 – 3 seeds in each berry, a couple hundred of mature healthy plants can easily provide you with a pound of green seed.

Some growers will choose not to harvest berries from their mature plants in favor of encouraging faster root growth. This requires removing the berry stalk when the clusters emerge as small flowers early in the growing season. Thus by carefully removing the berry-prong the energy that would have gone towards the berries will be invested into the plant and more importantly the root.

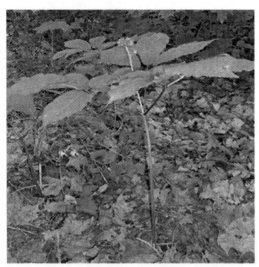

Mature Ginseng Plant with Flowers Developing into Berry Cluster

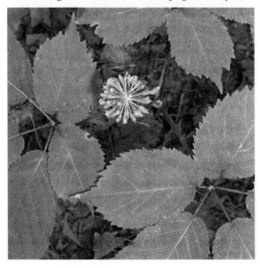

(i) De-pulping Harvested Seed

Ginseng berries when properly harvested from a garden are normally de-pulped. When you have successfully grown a crop yielding berries be sure to check on the plants daily from the middle of August until the berries are fully ripened and the plants die back. The individual berries within a plant's cluster will not be ready all at once and other predators will gladly collect them if they are left on the plant for long. You should get into the habit of always having Zip-loc plastic bags with you for storing fresh berries that are harvested when inspecting the gardens in late summer.

Upon berry removal from the gardens and returning back to your house, either place the seeds in plastic bags in the refrigerator until you are ready to de-pulp them or proceed to de-pulping. If the berries are being stored in the refrigerator with their pulp try not to let them be stored for more than a couple of weeks.

To de-pulp, place the berries in a bucket and squeeze them with your hands. Work through the berries until the pulp is gently removed off from the seeds. Then slowly add water to the bucket so the pulp will float to the surface above the seeds remaining in the bottom, repeat several times until the pulp is fully separated from the seeds. Next place the seeds in a safe environment to prevent them from drying out. At this point it is best to store seeds in the refrigerator until you have a large enough quantity collected to place them into a box to stratify.

Therefore store the de-pulped seeds in a Zip-loc type bag in the refrigerator, not sealed airtight but 95 percent sealed and rolled on itself. If your seeds will be in refrigeration for more than a couple of days, on every second day pull out the plastic bags, open them up, and move the seeds back and forth with clean hands allowing fresh air to circulate in among them.

While storing the seeds in the refrigerator make sure people in your house are aware of them, and what they are, so that the seeds do not end up accidentally being discarded.

If you have modest gardens and a limited seed yield, it is likely easier to just leave the collected berries in plastic bags in the refrigerator until all ripe berries from all gardens have been collected for that season (it may take 2 – 3 weeks before all of them become ripe) then de-pulp those and place them into stratification together.

(ii) Stratification

Ginseng in its natural cycle needs to complete a period of stratification while the embryo of the seed is prepared for germination. Since ginseng seeds go through this 19 - 21 month period from ripe berry to yearling in a suspended state of cool then warm temperatures, green seed either harvested or purchased needs to be stratified. The best way to do this is in a controlled stratification box.

While your seed is safely in the refrigerator, build a stratification box out of wood. The size of the box and how many you construct will be predicated on how much seed you plan on stratifying. It is far better to make several smaller boxes rather than trying to make one large one, so keep the ones you make a manageable size.

As for building material, choose boards of regular lumber such as pine or other scraps (watch out for paint or pressure treatment if you are aiming for organic ginseng). The size of the boards comprising the box ideally should be from material that is ½ inch thick by about eight inches wide. Thus your cut boards will create a box eight inches high, but these are just suggestions if your lumber stock that is readily available is 10 inches wide then that will work as well. Nail or screw the boards together so that they make a box that is about 10 x 10 inches. Next, staple aluminum screening to the bottom of the box frame so as to have about one staple every inch (with the screen use aluminum so it will not rust). Screening size should be about the gage of standard window screening, for it to be ideal.

Then have ready several pounds of fine sand, the type that can be purchased at any garden store. Remove your seed from the refrigerator, and place the box (screen-side down) atop a firm piece of cardboard (this cardboard will keep the soon-to-be contents from sifting out through the screen). Apply a one-inch layer of sand into the box followed by a one-inch layer of seeds, then another inch of sand, then another inch layer of seeds and continue. When you are finished with adding layers of sand and seeds, fill the remainder of the box with sand.

Cut Away Look at Typical
Stratification Layering in an
Eight-Inch Deep Wooden Box

.........Screening-Top.....
2" Sand

1" Green Seed

1" Sand

1" Green Seed

1" Sand

1" Green Seed

1" Sand
.........Screening-Bottom.

At this point using staples, staple on a second screen to cover the top of the box. Staples are the choice better than small nails or tacks because you are going to eventually remove them to get to the seeds also use staple-gun staples because they are easier to remove than bottom staples.

Burying the box is the final step. Proceed to a pre-selected site that has suitable drainage. Keep in mind that this is only a holding-pen for your seeds thus if you are forced for lack of space to bury them under pines that is fine but an area shaded with hardwoods is better and good drainage is a must. Dig a hole deep enough so the top of the box will be three inches below the surface of the ground. The bottom of the hole must be scraped flat because this will help eliminate any air pockets underneath the box when it is buried. Upon completing the hole, have extra sand ready for burying your box. This is because when you place the box in the ground you will then pull the cardboard (it is easier if you have a protruding section to grab on to it) and as expected some sand will bleed through the bottom screen. Therefore have extra sand ready to pour into the box. Do not worry that your careful layering will be altered at this point it is not that critical. Thus after the cardboard removal, the added sand in the box should make it once again flush with the top screen. Now place a vertical marker stick on each side of the four sides of the box, allow the sticks to protrude up past the surface of the ground so that you will know the proportions of the box when it is buried. The soil that was removed from the hole is now filled in around the box. Use the excess soil to mound over the top of it, which helps protect the seeds by providing extra covering over the box. This modest mound also facilitates good drainage by helping to prevent water from gathering over the site which could otherwise settle and create a puddle over time. Furthermore the mound helps physically mark the area.

Then thoroughly document the spot, or spots if more boxes are sunk, into your logbook because one year can be a long time to remember the location among the many other things in life. It is easier to forget then you may think, especially in the woods where things quickly conform to a uniform look. Remembering the general area is not enough you will be looking for a buried 10 x 10 inch box, a relative needle in the haystack.

Next, fast-forward prior to planting, either one-year for the fall preceding the growing season or about 19 - 21 months if you are plucky and lucky enough to plant in the spring. Assuming everything progressed as planned, locate the box and very carefully dig it up. Be careful not to destroy the box or the bottom screening in the process with careless digging. This is why the sticks at the corners (or adjacent to the sides) marking the exact proportions of it work great.

Remove the box out of the hole carefully and bring it to a garden hose or an outside faucet. Preferably with a garden hose, rinse the box from the top, allowing the sand to trickle through the screening on the bottom. Keep working the water through. Once the sand is finally separated you remove the top screen and dump the seeds into a bucket. Add water to the seeds in the bucket until the mass bulk of seeds are submerged by several inches. The next step is the float test.

(iii) The Float Test

While your seeds are in the bucket submerged in water you conduct what is known as the "float test." This will show you what seeds have germinated. The seeds that float with the water level did not develop into seeds that are viable. Theoretically this does not have to be done to purchased stratified seed prior to planting because it is carried out by the sellers. At this point scoop off any that are floating and discard them. Then after the floaters are removed work your hand through the seed bulk in the bucket, freeing up any that may be at the bottom of the pile to make sure you remove all seeds that are not capable of germination.

After discarding the floaters, drain off your water and spread the seeds out on a screen or newspaper to air-dry for at least 10 minutes. Then collect the seeds to prevent them from drying out. For storage, the quart-size Zip-loc bags are very efficient. We find them exceedingly convenient and reliable. Therefore the next step is to zip the bag all the way shut (notice this time you want the seeds airtight) and folded on itself for storage in the refrigerator, unless you are immediately heading out to your prepared garden beds for planting. If the seeds are spending several days in the refrigerator, then once again, every several days shake the seeds around to let new air in, then after 2 – 3 minutes close the bag up. If you do not zip-up the bag completely the seeds readily dehydrate. We recommend one-cup of seed per bag, which averages around five ounces or 2500 seeds per Zip-loc. While these seeds are packaged keep them in the refrigerator (except for the occasional opening and airing them out) until your planting site is prepared and ready. The temperature in the refrigerator should be maintained between 35 – 40 degrees (Fahrenheit) and the seeds should not be allowed to freeze.

D) Cleaning Seed Before Planting

Whether you are planting new stratified seed, green seed, or removing the seeds you stratified yourself from the refrigerator, it is wise to clean them with a mixture that will kill disease on contact. This is a simple step and given how much work you have put into your gardens and will soon put into planting, it borders on insanity not to undertake this preventative measure unless you are an organic grower. Disinfecting seed has been broached earlier but here it is covered in greater detail.

Once you have reached the planting site and the gardens are prepared (or this step can be completed at home shortly before arriving to the gardens), you will be ready to plant right after you make a solution and mix it with the seeds. Create a solution of Manzate 200 with the measurements of 1-tablespoon to 1-gallon of water, for a smaller batch use ¼ tablespoon of Manzate 200 to a quart of water. Manzate 200 is an effective fungicide certified for use on ginseng.

After your solution is mixed (a washed-out plastic milk jug works well to mix it in) open the Zip-loc bags and pour in the Manzate solution so all seeds are covered. Set for 10 minutes, after 10 minutes un-zip the Zip-loc just enough to be able to dump the solution out without losing seeds. To aid with this, put a small twig in the corner of the zipper seal, then seal (or zip) the bag while the twig acts as a spacer preventing the seal from becoming watertight. Remove the twig then let the solution slowly drain emptying out the entire Manzate mixture.

Next from a clean jug of plain water, pour it into the bag to rinse off the Manzate 200 solution. Work the fresh water around the bag with your hands on the outside of it for about 20 seconds. Then using a twig as a spacer once again, open the bag, insert the twig, close it, and carefully dump the fresh water rinse out of the bag.

Growers can use a bleach solution for this cleaning step with the same directions as the Manzate 200. However we rather use the Manzate 200 instead of the bleach because we had a substantially lower germination rate with the bleach solution even trying different concentrations of both stronger (1 to 8 ratio) mixtures as well as weaker ones. Although those poor results may only be anecdotal, with growing ginseng one must find what works best and run with it. A third potential disinfectant mixture is made with Captan, but Captan is not really a fungicide so much as it protects the surface of the plants or roots with a coating. The proportions are 1-tablespoon of Captan to 1-gallon of water and then let the seeds soak for 10 – 15 minutes. After the solution is worked through the seeds, it is dumped out but you do not rinse the Captan solution off with fresh water like you would with the Manzate 200 or a bleach mixture. Also always be conscious of the chemicals you utilize and carefully discard them in an environmentally favorable manner. The Manzate 200 and Captan will be used in the garden anyway but you should be responsible where it ends up.

Whether you opt for the bleach, or Manzate 200 solution, after you have used it and rinsed the seeds with fresh water, then dumped them out on a sheet of newspaper to air-dry, allow them to sit for about 10 minutes.

At this point it is helpful to have the seeds air-dried because when wet they will stick to your fingers making planting tantalizing and frustrating. These seeds are small and weigh very little, like lentils. If you complete this disinfecting step at home, after 10 minutes place the seeds in a plastic container like a Tupperware or Coolwhip container but make sure the seeds are planted that day preferably within several hours.

E) Starting with Rootlets

Rootlets ordered through the mail should receive the same treatment with the Captan, bleach, or Manzate 200 solution that the seeds did. Also it is advisable to use this solution to clean rootlets transplanted or removed for quarantining. After they arrive in the mail, take them out of their packaging and conduct the disinfecting in the same manner as the seeds. Then plant as soon as possible, thus ideally your gardens will be ready and waiting. Beginners might find it fun to experiment with ordering rootlets along with seed, that decision is up to the grower. The best financial return is successfully starting from seeds and selling them as dried roots after their harvest. Rootlets offer a much more expensive initial investment but give the grower the chance to observe, own, and admire older plants from the outset.

Chapter VI

Threats and Risk Management

The role of limiting factors in plants and animals is believed by scientists to prevent domination and overpopulation and such factors like disease can be devastating. Whether it is in humans with pandemics, like the influenza outbreak that struck near the end of the Great War (1914 - 1918) killing conservatively an estimated 20 – 40 million people worldwide (compared to the estimated 8.5 million killed in four years of war), or in trees like the Dutch elm disease that began ravaging entire populations in the 1920s, disease occurs in nature and ginseng is also vulnerable. Disease is not the only risk to ginseng but it can be one of the most capricious literally decimating gardens in days. Therefore this chapter discusses the most dangerous fungi and animals that impact ginseng. There is also mention of the lesser miscellaneous threats that every grower needs to be aware of.

A) The Four Horseman of Ginseng Destruction

The four most common threats that will attempt to assail your crop are:
  (i)   Blight
  (ii) Dampening-Off
  (iii) Root Rot
  (iv) Animal Infiltration

The first three are diseases and we shall take a moment and discuss prevention. The old platitude of *an ounce of prevention is worth a pound of cure* certainly rings true with ginseng. Reasonable spraying and clean habits can substantially mitigate the potential of catastrophe. Although the diseases discussed in this chapter are not the entire list of potential pathogens that attack ginseng, they are the most common and preventing them will forestall the more obscure. Furthermore at some point these *Four Horsemen* will likely visit your crops because growing ginseng is a game of attrition. If you planted 7,500 seeds in the fall it is folly to assume that it will grow into 7,500 plants. Though it is hard to keep records on this you will at least loose 10 – 30 percent after the first growing season, but these losses are already planned for and anticipated. It is part and parcel of accepted risks. Three years later you may have to remove thirty plants to save several hundred in a garden, these lifeboat-ethics must be practiced to be a successful grower. Every seed will not become a plant and every plant cannot be saved, the *Four Horsemen* will take their toll but you plan for it while taking every precaution possible to avoid them.

All tools used for ginseng should only be used for ginseng or thoroughly cleaned before you begin using them to work on your gardens. We have our garden tools for ginseng painted white (red would also work) to help keep them separated from our regular shovels, hoes, hatchets, rakes, and pruners that are used around the house. The flat white color is also practical, in fact since painting them we have not lost or misplaced any of these tools in the woods, which is otherwise not hard to do during the hectic fall planting. Also if you use an implement to remove a diseased plant make sure it is cleaned before it goes back to the tool shed. Clean them in a 1 to 8 solution of bleach to water, then rinse them off with water.

Ideally when working in your gardens you should wear clothes and shoes that have not been in places that can track in disease such as barnyards, vineyards, orchards, or any foreign environment. It is well worth having one pair of rubber boots only for ginseng gardening. Never allow tobacco to be used near your ginseng, these products are notoriously replete with disease-causing organisms even after processing. Always use the pathways created in between your gardens so that you do not have to step into them, this is why the four feet garden-width is the standard to make it easy to reach into but not step into the garden where the plants are growing. Failing to disinfect new seeds and rootlets places you at risk. Dense planting increases the chances of disease as well and hastens its proliferation, which is why in the chapter on creating gardens we favor sparser planting rather than encouraging closer populations. Over fertilizing is another factor that can facilitate disease, the old saying *you cannot get something for nothing* is certainly true with ginseng. If you try to grow the plant too quickly, its immune system will suffer as well as the price of the root at auction since it will likely resemble the lower priced field cultivated variety. The field cultivated ginseng can survive the dense planting, accelerated growth, and inundation with fertilizer because it is heavily sprayed every week during the growing season.

With ginseng the lack of proper drainage can often be a major factor for disease. Proper drainage is paramount and part of the **SDS** formula (**Shade, Drainage, Soil**). Wet soggy soil is paradise to fungi that will devour your roots and quickly spread. Finally, plants under stress be it from too much sunlight, water, and nutrients, or too little, can be in a vulnerable state and unable to stave off disease that otherwise healthy plants are able to defeat. It all sounds like an impossible balance at first, but if you follow the directions set forth in this text you will likely have only isolated problems.

Spraying is one of the best habits you can adopt to keep your gardens healthy, green, and relatively disease free. The frequency is predicated on the weather, the density of your planting, as well as disease outbreaks. Although there is chatter in some scientific circles about eventually engineering disease resistant plants, that day is still far away.

The techniques and chemicals used with spraying are discussed in depth in the next chapter, (*see* Chapter VII

Spraying). For now we continue familiarizing you with the threats to ginseng.

(i) Blight
Alternaria
This leaf and stem blight is one of the most common and serious of the blights. The fungus responsible for it is *Alternaria panax*.

Signs
The otherwise healthy green-purplish stem that existed earlier in the season may take on orange-brown lesions as the plant collapses over. Also look for black spores on the affected area. If it is on the leaves they will develop dead, brittle, brownish lesions, also described by many as "papery" spots due to their thin crunchy consistency. Inspect these spots, if it is Alternaria they likely will have an irregular shape. They can be very asymmetrical, occurring in the middle of the leaflet or the edge. Look for the classic Alternaria-yellow halo or yellowish perimeter around the brown lesion.

How it Spreads
The Alternaria blight is caused by a fungus. This fungus likely will infiltrate your gardens by spores. The spores can be delivered in the wind, tracked in by an animal (or a human with spore-imbued clothes), implements, or shoes with the spores attached. Once the fungus settles in the garden it sits dormant in the mulch waiting for the right conditions like a rainy/humid stretch of weather when it can flourish and spread. Once established in your garden the spores can now spread through draining water, plant to plant contact, wind, or animal conveyance.

Results
The plant top eventually dies back but the root usually is not in danger although sometimes it can be affected. Alternaria

should not be underestimated, although your root most likely will survive only losing the rest of that growing season, it can spread among your plants with surprising speed.

Treatment

Once you have sufficient reason to suspect Alternaria, remove the plant top with extreme caution. Cut the top or tops off, place them in a bucket and quickly leave the garden, clean all implements and clothes that came into contact with the diseased plant or plants. When conditions during the summer, especially around thunderstorm systems, are conducive to fungi you should increase your spraying frequency. A maneb, Bordeaux mix, or preventative spraying with Captan will help contain minor Alternaria outbreaks. After an area is afflicted heavily douse the epicenter of the outbreak with a maneb or other suitable fungicide spray solution.

Prevention of severe outbreaks echoes the common themes. Increases airflow by removing all low lying branches not needed for shade. Air circulation helps dry the surface of the gardens reducing moisture and standing water, which otherwise creates conditions ideal for spores to grow and spread. Also under usual circumstances remove weeds that are restricting favorable airflow across the surface of the mulch. Furthermore gardens that are not planted dense allow air to pass between the plants as well as keeping afflicted plants from touching one another thus making an outbreak more difficult to spread. Usually if you spray responsibly, stay vigilant, and remove diseased plants when they occur, Alternaria will make only brief appearances throughout the growing season.

Botrytis

Botrytis is a less common blight in ginseng but one that is the same fungus that creates the gray mold on strawberries. It is attributed to the fungus *Botrytis cinerea* and can strike the leaflets, stems, roots, and berries. Look for the grayish velvety patches growing on your plants. If it is on a berry then carefully remove it. Good air flow around your gardens and copious removal of leaves, limbs, and other foreign debris that descend into them will help keep fungi and spore sanctuaries away from your plants. Spraying responsibly with fungicides preventing Alternaria blight will help prevent and control Botrytis. As usually the case with Alternaria leaf and stem blight, Botrytis will not kill the root.

(ii) Dampening-off
This condition usually will be found afflicting yearlings. It is brought on by cool and wet weather along with poor drainage early in the growing season. Dampening-off can be caused by the Alternaria fungus as well as these other culprits: *Phytophthora, Pythium, Fusarium, & Rhizoctonia*. It attacks the stem of the plant just above the soil. Several of the common fungi that cause dampening-off are already in the soil therefore it can strike a plant before it even gets a chance to break the surface. That condition is known as pre-emergence dampening-off.

Signs
If it strikes the plant look for a lesion on the plant stem that causes the yearling to flop over coupled with wet cool weather. Usually it will hit early in the growing season. Dampening-off does not seem to successfully destroy older plants as it does yearlings, the prevailing theory is that the older plants develop a resistance.

How it Spreads
The conditions in the environment and soil aiding this outbreak are an overly moist, wet, and damp ground. These factors may help the spores spread. Also densely planted yearlings help facilitate the spread of spores.

Results

Once afflicted a seed or yearling will subsequently die.

Treatment

The only way to really limit dampening-off is to continue with what by now is a familiar refrain, utilize raised beds with good drainage, proper airflow, and try not to plant too dense. Also never plant in a field where alfalfa was the prior crop if you are undertaking field cultivated ginseng unless you let the field stand for at least one year. The Rhizoctania fungus, finds alfalfa favorable, which can cause dampening-off in ginseng.

A proper pH helps promote healthy plants. Also keep your seed depth of ½ - 1 inch when sowing seed so that the plant does not exhaust its strength trying to break through the ground early in its growth.

Heavy mulch might exasperate the problem since fungi thrive in moisture and may prevent fungicide from trickling down to the soil surface, of course not enough may allow the soil to become too warm and dry thus hurting the yearlings. The best balance is struck by sensible mulching of ½ of an inch and responsible spraying of yearlings when they begin to emerge. Implementing proper preventative habits should vastly reduce dampening-off to a minor nuisance.

In the rare event that dampening-off hits a garden with fury, carefully peel back your mulch to the bare ground and heavily spray the garden with a concentrated maneb fungicide every three days and isolate the afflicted area with perimeter trenching (10 – 12 inches from the dying plants) because the fungus can spread underground from infected roots. You will need to strike a delicate balance, leaving the mulch off of the garden until the wet weather passes but not waiting until the soil becomes too dry. As soon as the conditions begin to dry, start covering the garden where the old mulch was with new mulch.

(iii) Root Rot

Unlike blights where the plant dies back but the root often survives, this is not the case with root rot. While Alternaria leaf blight can severely devastate your gardens for the season root rot will destroy them forever.

Phytophthora

The most common root rot cause is the fungus Phytophthora. Alternaria can cause root rot as well, along with the less common fungi: *Cylindrocarpon, Fusarium, Pythium,* and *Sclerotinia*. However Phytophthora remains the most serious. It is spread by water and is not initially airborne. Therefore it thrives in weather conditions of above average moisture, such as rainy/wet conditions. Though it really is a protist, it has fungus-like attributes and is grouped with them. The spores can be carried downhill in the draining rainwater of your garden, they can be conveyed via ricochets of rainwater bouncing off infected plants, plant to plant contact, and even by way of contact with a passing animal. Either you, a deer, or any other animal could spread these spores if they are attached

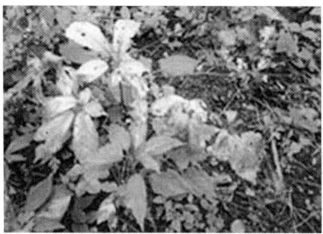

Phytophthora: Beware of Red & Yellowish
Colored Leaflets in Summer (above)

Alternaria Leaf Blight: Discoloration & Blotches on Leaflets
Displaying a Yellow Halo (below)

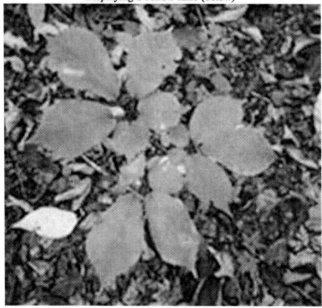

while walking through an infected garden area in the same
manner Alternaria leaf blight can spread. Mulch will help

reduce Phytophthora by preventing water from splashing spores onto your plants and regular spraying of systemics like: Aliette WDG, Dithane DF, Ridomil Gold, or copper sulfate (preferably in the Bordeaux mix-fungicide which is discussed in Chapter VII Spraying).

Signs

With the rot underground the only visible sign will be that the leaflets of the plant begin to display colored lesions very similar to Alternaria blight. Phytophthora often first manifests itself as a leaf and stem blight (known as Foliar Phytophthora). This includes spots that become reddish, yellowish, or brown before they turn translucent and the leaflets begin to wilt because nutrients are being starved from the roots. Look for leaves that appear as if they have been burned by an extreme frost. Healthy green leaf tissue separates the papery-brown-translucent lesions with a deep greenish-black border. Sometimes by striking late in the growing season the dying leaves of the diseased plants blend in with the regular look of healthy ginseng naturally capitulating for that growing season. This sets the stage for the outbreak the following year. The oospores spend the winter inside the root of the afflicted plant or surrounding ground awaiting the chance to spawn the zoospores, these are the spores that can carry the fungus to new plants. Phytophthora will thus spread again when the opportunity presents itself. These oospores can live in a garden for years, once you have experienced Phytophthora do not plant anything in that section again, let the forest reclaim it. You do not want to tear open the ground allowing the spores to escape. Some growers will use the area for goldenseal cultivation however if other suitable land is available then consider not to taking the risk.

The roots of the diseased plants will be brittle, dark tan (instead of healthy white), and watery. However unless one is to dig the roots that fall they may not realize this, especially if it strikes late in the year. If you were oblivious to the presence of the fungus and harvested your roots after the growing season, the roots will be discolored and become blackish-blue when dried in the infected sections. If bacteria invaded the soft core it may have a stench, and obviously have a greatly reduced commercial value. Also other more obscure root diseases can cause discoloration and rot within the root and all will greatly reduce its commercial value.

How it Spreads
The fungus that causes this potentially crop-killing disease appears naturally in the soil and is even common in soil. A scenario as mundane and seemingly innocent as a heavy downpour splashing the spores from the ground to the leaflet of your plant can start the chaos, or from water under the soil moving and carrying the spores from one root to another.

Results
Unlike Alternaria where the root often survives, Phytophthora is a death sentence once the root is infected. If the top of the plant is removed before the disease reaches the root then it should be fine but keep an eye on that area of the garden. You should error on the side of caution and carefully extract the roots since Phytophthora can spread at a mortifying pace.

Treatment
When an outbreak occurs act immediately and carefully. Remove the afflicted ginseng as well as healthy-looking plants in a radius of 3 - 5 feet from the diseased plant or patch, even if they appear healthy. If possible partition this piece of garden with a trench having a depth of 8 - 10 inches. Lifeboat ethics come into play, better to risk killing 30 healthy-looking but potentially diseased plants than risk loosing thousands. That may sound dramatic but it can and will happen if a grower does not act fast. This is where your small isolated quarantine-garden beds come into use. If the surrounding plants look healthy they

still should be removed as a buffer from the main garden. If you are a gambler then remove their tops, bathe them in a Manzate 200 solution (1-tablespoon Manzate to 1-gallon of water) and place the roots in the quarantine bed of the otherwise healthy looking plants. The hope is that the Manzate will kill the spores on contact, be sure if the root is already surreptitiously infested it will not only perish but spread the disease, however in a quarantine bed, sparsely planted, it may not spread any further. With some luck they will emerge again next year safe, if they were diseased then nothing is lost but some time. Make sure you heavily douse the area that you removed the plants from with fungicide and clean everything that came into contact with the disease. Treat anything removed from that area as being toxic. Soil and visibly diseased roots should be removed far from your gardens. Your boots, tools, bucket, and anything else used in the extrication operation should be cleaned in a 1 to 8 bleach to water solution, and rinse with water.

Other more obscure root diseases can cause discoloration and root expiration but the precautions taken in the section on spraying and the aforementioned policy on quick removal of plants that look suspiciously sick should arm you with enough knowledge to stave off any serious setbacks.

Grower's Tip!

Look for spots or suspicious shapes because minor leaflet discoloration can be caused by many simple things for example: over spraying, too much sun, poor soil, insects, or abrasions caused by something foreign. If your plants begin to display red, yellow, watery, spots on the leaflets look for the classic elongated blemishes with the yellow halo on the perimeter, at this point you may be relatively *lucky* if it is "only" Alternaria, which offers this halo signal. If you proceed optimistically and assume that it is Alternaria blight keep a careful watch over that section of garden and increase the spraying frequency, although leaf sprays only kill on contact they can greatly reduce the spread.

If you notice the condition spreading with autumn hues on the leaflets like yellows and reds, (especially without the distinct yellow halo) then quickly assume the worst and remove the plants. Years ago we had a terrible attack of Phytophthora demolish a garden of wunderkind plants. They were a crop that had offered seed in their second year, they were tall, green, healthy, and appeared to be much older than they actually were without having been fed any fertilizer. One July with above normal rain, crushing humidity, and staggering heat, we noticed some suspicious colors in this garden of super-plants. It began at the bottom of the hill, which was separated by a new trench. We were foolish not destroying the contingency of diseased plant tops in the beginning. Within days, first dozens, then hundreds, then thousands of plants were in the throes of Phytophthora. Soon all but a handful, were vanquished. Therefore although instinct may force you to recoil at removing plants until you know they are indeed a threat, Phytophthora is not to be taken lightly. Far better to remove 50 plants that may or may not survive in the quarantine bed than leave them to spread the disease killing hundreds.

Rusty Root

Another root rot that is less common is called rusty root, so called because the root takes on a reddish brown corky composition, contrasted with the watery attributes of Phytophthora. The disease often begins at the tips and spreads slowly through the root. It does not usually kill the root but significantly reduces the commercial value of the ginseng. Unlike Phytophthora, the root will be corky not soft. Rusty root may exist without your knowledge because although sometimes it will engender orange or red discoloration to the leaflets, it does not have to. Rusty root is a slow moving disease and usually afflicts plants that are in their second growing season or more.

Once again cure by prevention. Rusty root is caused by a fungus, usually the culprit is *Cylindrocarpon destructans*. It appears in the soil naturally, which is usually present where ginseng has already grown. Keep tools and all other objects that have worked in a garden clean (with the 1 to 8 bleach to water solution, then rinse with water) after use. Try to plant roots sparse (one or two every square foot) when possible. Also try not to recycle ginseng beds, especially if you are planting with the field cultivated method or planting dense woods-grown crops. Woods-grown growers in the southern areas of the United States have not reported as many complications with replanting in the same site as growers in the northern United States and Canada have experienced. Usually it is better to replant a bed that yielded a healthy crop of ginseng with goldenseal as opposed to risking another ginseng crop. The method of rotating to goldenseal is covered later (*see* Chapter IX Growing Goldenseal).

Mystery Seedling Disease

Known as MSD, this is a lesser-known disease and may be a phase related to the previously mentioned, rusty root. It possibly could be the cause of seeds failing to grow or it may affect the plant during the growing season. Inspect the roots of yearlings after the growing season if the leaves displayed a red tinge. If upon inspecting the root it has a dark tan, decayed, almost mangled looking taproot and is shaped more like a bulb than the conventional long white carrot-shaped yearling root, you may have MSD.

Its cause is linked to several fungi possibly working in consort including: *Septonema*, *Fusarium*, *Pythium*, *Cylindrocarpon destructans*, and *Rhizoctonia*. Once it afflicts the root it seems to progress until the root dies. Much like rusty root, try to maintain cleanliness, create new gardens instead of replanting in areas previously harvested, clean tools and implements regularly with the 1 to 8 bleach to water solution, and avoid if possible importing soil into your beds. To the field cultivators, be sure to carefully disinfect any soil that is brought in with the proper chemicals.

(iv) Infiltration by Animals and Pests

When a healthy and mature ginseng plant has its berries turn from green to red, they stand out stark against the forest undergrowth especially on a plant that has leaves turning yellowish-green and dying back for the year. Deer, chipmunks, turkeys, raccoons, squirrels, rabbits, and humans need to be kept away from plundering your berry crop and plants. All animals in general can be dangerous to ginseng, walking through your gardens can break the stem of the plant destroying growth for that season or forever if it is a yearling, while potentially also tracking in disease.

As for humans, the old World War II phrase reminding people to keep from giving out secrets accidentally to the enemy applies-*loose lips sink ships*. If you are growing ginseng then keep it secret, no more than those who actively help you need to know of your operation. Some large-scale growers employ guard dogs and security cameras but responsible observation will suffice for most people to keep trespassers away. Despite the temptation, never set booby-traps or recklessly create conditions that could kill or seriously injure a potential vandal these are illegal in every jurisdiction in the United States.

Reduce the prevalence of other animals by harvesting your berries as they become red. It will not be all at once so make a point to get to your gardens at least every other day for the several weeks when they begin to ripen. As mentioned earlier if you do not remove the berries, other animals will do it for you. To scare birds and spook deer constructing simple scarecrows with arms that can flail in the wind may help.

Deer

Depending on where you live the local populations of deer can be very destructive. They will chew on ginseng plant-tops and make a mess by walking into the gardens throughout the growing season. In 2005, the journal of the American Association for the Advancement of Science offered an article predicting that wild ginseng could become extinct in areas of Appalachia within 100 years. This report attributed the devastation to deer grazing on the tops of the plants if they continue to do so at the current pace.

Threat Eradication

Although some growers put up fences this option was neither economically or practically feasible for our operation. The classic methods to repel deer involves hanging aluminum pie tins from low limbs as well as placing deodorant soap bars in nylon stockings and hanging them from nearby brush or trees. One other deer repellent that is worth trying is a mixture of Blood Meal, water, and ammonia.

The Recipe Requires:
1-Bucket of Water
2½ -Pounds of Blood Meal
1-Cup of Ammonia
Several Cubes of *Green Oasis* used for flower arranging or non-chemically treated Sponges will suffice

First combine the Blood Meal with the water in a bucket. Then add the ammonia. You will dip the cubes of cut Green Oasis or sponge into the solution and place them accordingly throughout the perimeter of the garden. These cubes can be simply attached to sticks or switches by stabbing them, then dipped into the solution, dip the cubes weekly into the solution.

The natural balance of nature may help as well. The more we expanded our ginseng operation the more welcome fox and coyotes were on our land. Both enjoy feasting on mice, and coyotes help with not only deer but also keeping the smaller pests like rabbits, raccoon, turkeys, and woodchucks away. Thus coyotes are always welcome in our woods.

Mice and Moles

Of the animal threats, it is likely that rodents will cause you the most problems. Moles like to tunnel into the garden beds and mice like to utilize these tunnels raiding roots as they come across them. The moles do not eat the ginseng as they are after insects in the soil but your gardens will be loose, rich, soil and moles easily can create a vast tunnel system in a relatively short period opening the door to mice and allowing too much air to get to the roots, which can also damage them. The mice will eat and plunder seed as well as small roots. While the larger roots are left in the garden the mice will eat on them, significantly damaging the root and its potential value.

Threat Eradication

Unfortunately although the moles are technically innocent they create the problem and must be removed with the mice.

Moles:

For the moles most garden stores or online gardening supply companies sell poison pellets for them that need only be dropped in their holes. For the organic growers, bubble gum also works well. The best option is to go to the bulk food section of your local supermarket and buy the small, cheap, pink, bubble gum, and place it in the mole holes. Cover them with a small flat stone, after about three days check the hole and step on it collapsing the tunnel.

Mice:

Traditional traps are easily sprung in the woods therefore the best treatment for these plunderers is poison. The trick is to keep the poison dry and only accessible to the mice. This can be accomplished easy enough by building some feeders out of PVC pipe. At a hardware store purchase some small diameter 1½-inch pipe that a mouse or vole could crawl into. There are two ways to go from here. The easy way is to then cut the pipes into 15

– 20 inch pieces and horizontally place them in promising spots around the garden. After that, anchor these pieces down with heavy rocks placed atop them. Then with a spoon or other device shovel the bait into the pipe-traps.

The second method is more work initially, but in the long run will prove to be much easier. First envision what you are building. A large inverted PVC "T" that will contain poison to kill mice. When buying the PVC pipe, stick with the 1½-inch diameter pipe stock. Proceed to separate the pieces into sections about two feet long. At a 45 degree angle (these will work as awnings against rain) cut the two-foot pipe in the middle at the 12-inch mark. After this you now have two pieces, each piece of pipe has a flush cut end and a 45-degree-cut end. Now plug the flush end into a "T" fitting making sure that when the trap is lying on the ground the 45 degree angel end will allow the extended edge to act as the awning. Add what will be the vertical piece of PVC, also measuring about 12-inches in length (you can make this longer if you wish), then glue the pieces together.

After the glue has dried you will have your trap but also a vertical shoot that will easily allow replenishing of the poison. Anchoring these traps can get tricky. A good place is near a tree where rocks can be placed on the horizontal pipe and more importantly the vertical portion can be safety-wired around an adjacent tree trunk. This vertical pipe section needs to be covered, which can be accomplished with a simple tin soup can.

Slugs and Snails

Slugs and snails are not covered under insects because they are mollusks. They should be destroyed at every opportunity. These culprits live in and below the mulch. Above the ground they feast on ginseng seed, stems, and any part of the root that may be showing even the bud for next year's growth. Sometimes if you have yearlings being devastated it may be slugs attacking the stems rather than dampening-off or some other fungus. They love the moist, damp, forest areas, and general habitat created by ginseng gardens. Also they remain active the entire growing season and in all weather systems, especially during a drought.

Threat Eradication

As menacing as they are, this problem is easily solved with slug bait that can be broadcast in the form of pellets. One of the best currently on the market is by the brand Deadline. Simply broadcast them over your gardens where the bait will usually remain for several weeks in pellet-form unless excessive rain dissolves them. Any garden store should carry slug pellets, for medium to large growers the big bags of 50 pounds should be acquired. Since they are a seasonal product (at least in the Northeast) you need to satiate your projected supply needs in the spring. Any extra pellets remaining store for the next growing season thus it never hurts to buy more supply than needed. Also it is worth calling around to different suppliers if you are in a rural area, you may get lucky and purchase them from a company that already delivers to local golf courses or farms thus saving on the expense of shipping costs.

An effective non-chemical solution is always the preferred method with ginseng, though not always the most practical. We try to keep several organic gardens just to experiment with. In these gardens we utilize non-chemical slug traps that were developed long ago by enterprising gardeners and they seem to work quite well for small plots.

The first is the most basic. It requires several sets of boards (make sure they are not pressure treated if you are vying for a truly organic environment). In spots around the gardens place one board on the ground, and sprinkle a dozen or so pebbles for spacers on it. Then place another board over the one on the ground, so that the pebbles are sandwiched between both boards. On the following morning, remove the top board and the pebbles, then place the top board back onto what should be a collection of slugs and proceed to squish them. Surprisingly leave the dead bodies mutilated on the board for the next night these will call more slugs and snails.

Traps for sale at garden stores or online are great but you can also make your own. The most well known is the *beer trap*. It simply requires a shallow container or pan sunk half of its depth into the ground with holes in it. For example take a Cool Whip or other small dairy container and carefully cut one-inch squares every 2 – 3 inches around the side that will be used as doorways for the slugs. The bottom of these cut squares should be about 1 - 2 inches from the bottom of the actual container. This is so the door-openings will be flush with the ground when the trap is sunk about 1 – 2 inches into the ground. Have a top handy that can be taken off with little ease. This will help keep debris and rainwater from diluting the bait. With the hole dug, and trap placed into it, then pour the beer into the container. The aroma will call the slugs, like the Sirens in Greek Mythology, to their destruction. Like the board trap, leave the dead bodies in the solution since it will call other hungry slugs. Every 2 – 3 days is a good duration in between dumping the trap since by then the beer will lose its strength. If you recoil at the thought of wasting beer for this, there is an alternative that may be cheaper.

In a Solution Mix:
2-Tablespoons of all Purpose Flour
½-Teaspoon of Brewer's Yeast
1-Teaspoon of Sugar
2-Cups of Warm Water
Snails and Slugs will find this Solution just as alluring as Beer.

B) Miscellaneous Threats

Insects
Insect infestations are usually not a major problem. There will be some small eating on leaflets by insects other than slugs that

at first resemble round tiny brown Alternaria spots (remember Alternaria usually produces elongated brown spots with a yellow perimeter). Some geographic regions have more insect problems than others. Warmer areas may see root knot nematodes their larvae live in the soil. They are microscopic and attack the root thus sometimes causing wilting and reddish discoloration of the plant. On the root the nematodes dwell in small wart-like bumps, which can be removed before the roots are sold. Ginseng can also be attacked by other insects like aphids and jumping plant lice, which grow on the flower stem resulting in what looks like dehydrated berries. The insects that do attack ginseng can usually be eradicated by using an insecticide that can be applied as needed with your regular summer spray routine (*see* Chapter VII Spraying).

Replant Disease

This is the phenomenon of drastically decreased yields when ginseng is planted in a plot that previously held a garden until harvest. Research has not adequately done more than identify the problem, which likely has many causes.

Disease Imposters

Disease is not always the culprit altering the color of the plants. Too much sunlight will cause discoloration, observe your garden during the day perhaps there is a hole in the canopy that you missed when assessing the garden previously or it may have just formed due to a branch dying. Too much water, too little water, or too much spraying can facilitate questionable blemishes. First take note of the spots on leaflets then consider the weather conditions, analyze the amount of spraying done and look for residue of any fungicides on the plants if any.

During relatively dry conditions, often cautiously waiting several days will be the adequate response to light minor discoloration. However remember that if the spots expand and a yellowish halo-perimeter appears around the worsening areas it likely is Alternaria and if a water blister-type lesion occurs with autumn colors then that is likely Phytophthora in either case at this point act swiftly and prudently.

Drought

It is sometimes easier to deal with a drought than a continual rainy weather pattern. Healthy and mature ginseng plants should easily survive a summer with sporadic arid periods. Actual drought conditions can be more serious and if they strike, depending on the severity, an irrigation project may need to be undertaken. The logistics will differ vastly with each grower. If you have ponds near the gardens, then a water pump powered by a gas engine and hose with an attached nozzle-sprayer may be all that is needed. Another economical option is to purchase some large water tanks (e.g. 275-gallon size) at a farm auction. Once these are filled with water and secured on an adequately constructed conveyance (like a decommissioned manure spreader) they can be taken right to the garden and delivered to the plants by a gas powered water pump and hose. An irrigation exercise can be time-consuming but usually not necessary unless you live in an environment prone to substantial seasonal drought.

An unfortunate result of a sustained seasonal drought upon mature plants that you may encounter is the reduction of the berry crop. In this situation the berry prong develops and even may produce some berries but the majority of the berries in the cluster are tiny, undeveloped, or practically nonexistent.

Chapter VII

Spraying

Supplies needed:
1) Sprayer
2) Fungicides
3) Spreader Sticker
4) Insecticide
5) Empty plastic containers
6) Small gage wire
7) Systemics
8) Small funnel
9) Rubber gloves
10) Water

From the previous chapter on the *Four Horsemen* and other risks we established that there are plenty of things that can be done without chemicals to try and prevent a disease outbreak. However comparing our organic gardens and regular gardens the results make it clear that a spraying routine will vastly increase the amount of plants that survive and make it to harvest while substantially facilitating disease containment along the way.

When undertaking spraying there are a couple of issues that must be sorted out. First the Environmental Protection Agency (hereafter EPA) has limited that which is legal to use on ginseng. Secondly you must check with the rules and regulations promulgated by your state environmental agency as well. Depending on the regulations in your state you may need to obtain an applicator's licenses to purchase certain chemicals. The Internet has made this sort of information gathering much easier. A link from the respective homepage of each state should direct one to its environmental agency and contact information. However if you are more comfortable with talking to someone, then look in the government section of your telephone directory for the local county extension of the Department of Agriculture they should be able to instruct you on how to obtain a copy of the regulations of your state and answer any questions. Furthermore a call to the local garden or agriculture supply store can often answer many questions as you can discover what chemicals are available to you.

A) Technique

Spraying is best accomplished with a backpack sprayer unless you have vast areas available and corresponding gardens to utilize the large tow-behind style. Since you are the creator of your gardens, the style of sprayer employed can be planned in advance. For our operation a four-gallon backpack sprayer is fine, it has a handle-activated agitator that keeps the mixture in suspension and is easy to manage when filled to three gallons.

This will be the most consistent labor-intensive aspect of growing in between preparing your gardens and harvesting the roots nonetheless even proceeding at a slow pace, several hours should be plenty of time to get the job done. When spraying your plants with a fungicide, be sure to reach the tip of the applicator up underneath the plant getting all parts of the stem and leaflets aside from just topical spraying. Maintain good pressure and a suitable spray. Do your best to avoid having the tip of the applicator touch the plants because this could damage the tissue of the leaflets making them vulnerable to later attacks. For disease prevention, even though you are spraying fungicides, always strive to keep physical contact with plants to a minimum.

(i) Frequency

With close planting such as yearlings in a seedbed, field cultivated, or dense woods-grown planting, during the growing season spray topical leaf fungicides weekly. For sparser planting every 10 – 14 days should be satisfactory if no problems are found in your garden. The fungicides you employ will last the indicated duration that they are effective, some will last longer than others, this specific information can be found on their labels. Most last about 7 – 10 days, but during an average summer of dry weather with reasonably generous spacing between plants, waiting two weeks in between spraying healthy gardens is satisfactory. Naturally this can all change in an instant if weather conditions become humid and wet, then it is necessary to spray weekly.

You will need to increase spraying if your plants begin to display signs of disease such as reddish, brown, yellowish leaflets unless you are causing damage with the chemicals. Over spraying can sometimes cause blemishes that may look like disease. One thing that will be obvious is if a leaflet has any chemical residue on it. The spreader sticker works on a molecular level to keep the fungicide on the leaves this diaphanous coating can be easily seen while it lasts because it offers a slight tint. Use deductive reasoning, if the weather has been dry, and you have been spraying every seven days, and the plants clearly still have fungicide on their leaflets, and you see some small isolated blemishes on a leaflet, then it may only be a burn mark from excessive spraying. Compared to experiencing rainy weather accompanied with heavy moisture and dense heat, even while spraying weekly under these conditions, if blemishes begin to develop always hope for the best but assume the worst when plants begin to display discoloration. The key is to prudently monitor the gardens and employ caution balanced with common sense.

While experiencing a rainy spell, you will have to spray with more frequency, this can be vexing if you spent the better part of the day spraying and two days later a series of thunderstorms dispense 1 - 2 inches of rain. Nonetheless several hours spraying will be less annoying than dealing with an Alternaria or Phytophthora outbreak and the subsequent loss of thousands of plants. Rain will wash the chemical from the plants eventually (even if applied with a spreader sticker) but the fungicide also breaks down naturally. Therefore the spraying frequency is less rigid and more fluid fitting the demands of a given situation. If you are worried then error on the side of caution and spray every 7 – 10 days until you find the best schedule.

B) Mixing the Solution

The mixture that is applied will have two roles. There are the fungicides that kill on contact and remain on the plant with the help of the spreader sticker for about a week. Then there are the systemics that are absorbed by the root and plant to fight disease from the inside. Both serve separate and important purposes. Throughout the growing season usually you will spray fungicides every 10 – 14 days but also a systemic like Ridomil twice a growing season once in the beginning and once at the midway point, unless like Benlate or Alliette the systemic chosen needs to be reapplied every few weeks.

First read the labels of the chemicals your purchase, make sure they list ginseng as EPA approved and make certain the state you are living in does not impose further restrictions. In many states the needed fungicides can be purchased in a garden store in others you will need to obtain an applicator's license.

These fungicides and systemics are chemicals, in some cases carcinogenic, and thus should be properly handled. It is advisable to spray with a raincoat in order to prevent the solution from being absorbed into the skin especially while operating the backpack-style sprayer. It is also wise to wear dishwashing gloves. Finally wash yourself thoroughly after applying the spray solution. It is better to exercise caution than risk overexposure. If you hire workers make sure they understand the potential dangers as well. You have a moral and legal duty to provide them with protective equipment and safe working conditions.

The labels often describe mixtures for large crops in ounces and gallons to be applied. For a small or medium grower it is immensely helpful to know that 1-level tablespoon per 1-gallon equates to 1-pound per 100-gallons. This is the common ratio with ginseng spraying, 1-tablespoon to 1-gallon, which has been encountered in earlier chapters.

For mixing purposes it is helpful to have some empty plastic gallon jugs and several five gallon plastic tanks available as well as the tank attached to your sprayer pre-marked with a permanent marker, linier marks or lines delineating the amount of liquid per gallon works best. Some tanks are labeled or feature embossed plastic numbers but for those that are not, fill it with a gallon of water and mark it with a permanent felt-tipped marker, add a second gallon and mark that, and so on. This will greatly increase efficiency later. Some chemicals are liquid but many are in powdered form either way you will need to take your chemicals, sprayer, and extra water (in the tanks and jugs) to your gardens and any simple trick that makes measuring in the field quicker and easier is worth adopting.

Example of Making a 3-Gallon Mixture During the Growing Season

1) Add ½ of the water for the amount of spray you want to mix, in our example of an average mid-summer mix of 3-gallons that would be 1½-gallons of water added.

2) Add 3-tablespoons of chemical powder fungicide (i.e. Manzate 200), if instead of Ridomil you choose a systemic requiring application more often like Benlate then at this point also apply 3-tablespoons of that chemical to the mix. Close the sprayer tank and shake the contents for several minutes to help dissolve the fungicide and systemic with the water.

3) Add the remaining amount of water, which in this example is 1½-gallons.

4) In a separate container (like a cleaned soda bottle) mix and dissolve about 1-tablespoon of spreader sticker and 1-cup of water, then dump this into the tank with the existing 3-gallons of solution and shake the tank again mixing the contents up.

Grower's Tip!
Take note that water weighs about eight pounds to the gallon. In the previous example a three gallon solution is 24 pounds before factoring in the weight of the sprayer, obviously if this is too heavy or awkward then make smaller mixtures. It also helps when spraying to slosh the solution in the tank by rocking sideways every now and again to help keep the contents in suspension since most pump agitators can only do so much. It may look silly but it is far less aggravating than dealing with a clogged spray nozzle.

(i) Systemics
These chemicals are the only way to prevent disease from inside the plant, unlike topical fungicides that remain on the exterior. Depending on the type of systemic, some last much longer than regular fungicides like Ridomil, which can last 60 days and others only half that or even less like Benlate previously discussed, however both systemics and leaf fungicides are needed for a balanced spray routine.

Ridomil 2E is one of the best to help combat Phytophthora, which causes root rot as well as dampening-off. Ridomil needs to be carried down into the soil with rainwater where the roots can absorb it. Therefore a spreader sticker is not employed and it should be sprayed early in the spring shortly before an expected heavy rain. Only apply Ridomil once at the beginning of the season if a garden will be harvested that fall. Otherwise give the regular gardens a second dose at the midway mark. Since Ridomil will be applied in a heavier than usual spray and no spreader sticker is used, it is best to not try and apply a fungicide along with the typical twice per season application of Ridomil. Besides, Ridomil should be sprayed before a rainstorm, preferably a rain that will bring at least ½ of an inch of rain, contrasted to the other sprays that should be applied after a rain has passed.

Two other excellent systemic chemicals are Aliette 5G and Benlate 50 DF (DF translates to dry flowable powder). Aliette is absorbed into the leaves and increase the natural abilities of the plant to fight disease. Before being absorbed it kills fungi on contact on the exterior of the plant. Benlate is absorbed through the leaflets and lasts about two weeks and it will help prevent dampening-off along with root rot.

(ii) Fungicides

Topical leaf fungicides are helpful because they kill on contact. This may not sound like enough protection but it works extremely well when in balance with a proper spray routine and a spreader sticker. The spores are killed on contact, then the fungicide remains on the leaflets and stem for a week or so depending on the ability of the fungicide before it naturally breaks down its preventative barrier.

The most common and arguably effective family of fungicides to use is the manebs. The full name is manganous ethylene-bisdithiocarbomate, there are various brands by different manufactures but we use Manzate 200 for convenience and habit. If you find a better and cheaper maneb that offers the same attributes as Manzate 200 then feel free to experiment. Manzate remains on the plant about a week and can be observed with the goldish tint that it imbues the surface of the leaflets with and overall works very well at fighting the spread of blights.

If the spores of a fungus have already breached the surface tissue of the leaflet or stem a contact fungicide like a maneb will not be able to prevent further internal spread. This is why systemics and fungicides are kept up because they both have their own advantages as well as limitations.

Captan is another chemical that can be sprayed. It is really more of a shield that is applied. Not being a maneb it cannot be expected to kill fungus on contact, instead it leaves a coating on the plant in theory preventing fungus from attaching itself to the plant. Captan will last 10 – 14 days but is somewhat tame compared to a maneb however it is reputed to help fight dampening-off.

(iii) Spreader Sticker

Spreader sticker helps disperse the solution onto the leaves and stems. Furthermore it prevents modest amounts of moisture from washing the mixture off from the plants before it has the chance to naturally breakdown. Commercial spreader sticker should be added to fungicides but not a systemic like Ridomil that needs to be carried down to the roots. The spreader sticker on the market today is safe, relatively inexpensive, and easy to obtain. A few people may recommend using dishwashing soap as a spreader (but it is not a sticker) or other obscure additives. Avoid these if possible and stay with spreader sticker. These spray chemicals are relatively expensive and the spreader sticker works well and also is fairly cheap. Therefore there is little reason to experiment with the lesser quality spreader sticker techniques.

(iv) The Bordeaux Mix

This was developed in the Bordeaux region of France for use on their extensive grape crops. Eventually this innovative fungicide made its way to America. The Bordeaux mix has been attributed with not only fighting the common ginseng blights, but also the dreaded root rot fungus of Phytophthora. This can be a bit controversial because there is a chance that the Bordeaux mix may be illegal in your state to use on ginseng, which is unfortunate because it is one of the most economical, effective, and safe fungicides to apply. Of course a grower has the responsibility of checking local laws to learn what is legal and what is forbidden.

The issue with chemical regulations for ginseng and the government in general is epitomized with this issue. For a chemical company to obtain the right to list ginseng on their label as a crop that their chemical can be legally used on, the company undergoes a costly and time-consuming tolerance process. The process, among other things, gives the EPA the opportunity to make sure unsafe levels of chemicals will not reside in the roots or impact the surrounding environment. If a fungicide can be made by anybody for pennies on the dollar (like Bordeaux mix can if mixed yourself) then a company is not likely to sponsor the tremendous amount of resources needed to achieve governmental sanction for its use.

If you live in an area where there are no regulations against using the Bordeaux mix you will no doubt find it the favored fungicide. The containers used during the process of making Bordeaux mix cannot be made of metal. Only use plastic or glass, but plastic is far more practical. New plastic garbage cans work very well for this. Begin making the mixture at least one day in advance of using it.

To Mix a Medium Batch you will need:
2-Large Plastic Containers (like clean plastic garbage cans)
12½-Gallons of Water
3-Plastic Buckets
1-Pound of Copper Sulfate
1-Pound of Hydrated Lime
2-Simple Tools to use for Stirring the Mix

1) In the first large plastic container dissolve 1-pound of copper sulfate and 6¼-gallons of water. While mixing with a simple implement, you should find the copper dissolve quite readily. After stirring is complete, cover the container and let it sit for a day.

2) In the second large plastic container dissolve 1-pound of hydrated lime with the remaining 6¼-gallons of water. Using a different stirring implement than utilized with the copper sulfate, mix the lime. It will not dissolve as easy as the copper sulfate but give it a good vigorous stir before you cover it, and then let it also sit for a day.

3) After the passage of at least one day, and you are ready to spray, uncover the containers and with a different implement for each respective container mix them up again until the constituents

are in suspension. Especially watch the hydrated lime, it will need another bit of intense stirring.

4) It is IMPORTANT when mixing the two not to ruin the mixture, it will be a 50:50 ratio of copper sulfate solution to hydrated lime solution, but it must be combined carefully. It helps if in the smaller buckets a felt-tip permanent marker has been used to mark different volumes, such as a 1 - 1½ -gallon mark. At this point take a smaller bucket and scoop out the amount of hydrated lime solution that you desire to use, now with a second bucket SLOWLY pour in the same amount of copper sulfate into the hydrated lime solution, stirring the combined solution as it is poured into the bucket containing the hydrated lime. At this juncture, if the mixtures are not combined together correctly, the solution will curdle and if attempted to be used will clog the nozzle of the sprayer.

5) With the two solutions combined, congratulations you now have Bordeaux mix. As you pour the Bordeaux mix into the tank of the sprayer use a nylon screen to help filter out the larger undissolved particles of hydrated lime and other debris to avoid the nozzle from plugging during spraying.

6) If you are spraying systemics (like Benlate or Alliette) along with the Bordeaux mix, simply dump in 1-tablespoon for every gallon of Bordeaux mix into the sprayer tank and 1-tablespoon of spreader sticker for 3-gallons of spray solution.

7) This mixture should be promptly used. HOWEVER the two large separate containers still holding the hydrated lime and copper sulfate solution if covered can last until it is used up or even all summer.

(v) Insecticides

Insecticides should only be used when necessary because they can kill beneficial critters. Insects seem to be more a regional issue than a uniform problem. The more common culprits are aphids, cutworms, jumping plant lice, tree crickets, and leafhoppers. Some signs may be small holes in the leaflets, damage to the skin on the berries, or a cottony clump attached under the berry cluster damaging the overall health and quality of the berries. Conventional ginseng insecticides are diazinon, malathion, rotenone, and pyrenone (organic). Most can be applied along with the regular spraying of fungicides but they should only be administered about 2 – 3 times a season.

(vi) Foliar Fertilizing with the Regular Spray Routine

As discussed in Chapter III, if you feel the plants are not growing at a reasonably acceptable rate add some foliar fertilizer like Miracle-Gro 15-30-15. After your fungicide mix is made, and the spreader sticker is dumped in (and perhaps a foliar-absorbed systemic if desired), the final touch is to add the fertilizer into the tank of the sprayer. Miracle-Gro offers the familiar 1-tablespoon to 1-gallon ratio, so in the typical three-gallon solution throw in three tablespoons of Miracle Gro and shake the whole tank and you are ready to spray.

It is of course important to stress that you should not try to force-feed the ginseng plants or you risk weakening them. Ironically the concept of spraying is to protect the plants but by over-feeding you may weaken them. Also field cultivated commercial operations are turning out thousands of pounds of force-fed roots and the price paid at auction has consistently fallen in contrast to woods-grown roots gaining value. If you are attempting woods-grown ginseng then the goal is to create healthy but not commercial-looking roots. Usually 1 – 3 applications throughout the summer should be satisfactory.

Grower's Tip!

Take small gage wire as part of your supplies when embarking on a spraying detail. This wire easily can clean the spray nozzle, which may clog with particles of the dry mix that did not completely dissolve. Also take extra containers of clear water to rinse out the tank or clean any spilled mixture from you body or vehicle. Cleaned plastic milk jugs work well and

1-gallon plastic vinegar or windshield washer fluid containers work even better because they are a stronger grade of plastic. When possible, try to buy liquid over powder chemicals because obviously they dissolve more readily.

Remember that spraying is a preventative measure. You must be proactive not reactive therefore a good plan is to spray a systemic early in the growing season just as the plants are peaking through the mulch and promptly continue with systemics and fungicides in prudent intervals.

(vii) Weed Killers

Using a weed killer with ginseng may not be legal in your state. If it is, then it is a good idea to have a smaller secondary sprayer only used for weed killing mixtures and clearly labeled for such use. There are plenty of stories where growers mix a batch of fungicide into a sprayer that unbeknownst to them was not adequately washed from its prior weed killing solution and it is subsequently sprayed on the ginseng. Due to dilution the damage may be minimal but why take the chance? Never use weed killer in an existing ginseng garden. If it is being used while preparing a new garden then use the weed killer on the plot at least a month before actual planting of the ginseng seeds or rootlets.

The best ways to clear weeds in an existing garden is to pull them by hand. For a potential garden the rototiller will do an excellent job removing weeds without needing the chemicals of a weed killer.

Chapter VIII

Harvesting and Selling

Harvesting, drying, and selling your crop is a very liberating experience. In a way it feels strange you have labored over and protected these roots for years and now it is time to put them into the stream of commerce to hopefully be used to enhance the health of a consumer. In that respect it is nice to be growing a crop that will be used to improve the well being of another, and the financial return of a successful crop is also nice. How long you wait to dig your roots is your own accord but once removed from the ground it is important that you have a system in place whereby in the same day they can be carefully extracted, washed, and placed into drying. Of course this can be done one garden per day if need be, just prepare your room for drying ahead of time.

A) How Long Until Harvest?

The length of time to wait is predicated on growing methods and your sense of adventure. Field cultivated and highly fertilized ginseng, though in some cases three, can usually be harvested in four years. With the commercial methods your investment potential is in high volume selling and four years, maximum five years, is the duration to wait.

Woods-grown crops are a bit different because the health and size of a root is based on many variables. For instance the questions such as: did you apply fertilizer, remove the berry stalk early in each growing season (allowing the extra energy to be invested into the root), was the soil low in nutrients, did excessive shade (90 percent or more) stunt its development, all these need to be asked. An outstanding woods-grown crop can be ready for harvest in five years but 6 - 7 years is a more realistic average age of good quality dug roots.

During the growing season inspect the fullness of your 4 - 5 year old and older plants and their berry clusters (if you leave them on), when they are annually producing 30 - 40 fruits it is a good time to consider harvesting them. Eventually the root will reach a size whereby leaving it in the ground does not allow it to substantially grow any larger once it is producing these full berry clusters for a year or two. Although leaving them in the ground may bring in some substantial berry harvests, which can be sold or stratified, and the root may slowly gain slightly more weight, it is a prodigious gamble. If a natural disaster, disease, or human poacher were to strike, you would forever rue not harvesting when you could have and likely should have.

Those growers practicing wild-simulated will likely not find their plants suitable to harvest until 7 – 10 years depending on the growing conditions. The real sign like with woods-grown will be the appearance of the plant and its robust berry cluster. The root should weigh about an ounce before being removed from the ground. Should you accidentally dig a root that is too small and needs more growing time, quickly replant it without allowing it to dry out in the process and it should be fine.

(i) The Time of Year

The proper time to harvest ginseng is in the fall after the growing season and after the top has died back. At this point the root has received the fluid from the stalk and weighs its maximum while preparing for its winter dormancy. The only time ginseng should be harvested during the growing season is if severe disease or natural disaster compels you to extract it or face total loss and it cannot be transplanted to another area.

B) Digging the Roots

For large operations and field cultivated horticulturalists they will remove the structures supporting the artificial shade and then likely employ a mechanical digger. For the more modest growers extracting the roots by hand is the common practice. This step must be done carefully, damaging roots during harvesting would be a sickening mishap so take the time to brief any helpers on this matter and remember to only dig that which can be washed and prepared for drying that day.

While at the gardens begin by removing all mulch and loose plant tops. Your tool of choice can be a shovel, fork, spade, or any similar digging implement, but make sure it is cleaned before the digging is commenced. This is another example of where raised beds are advantageous making digging easier, but either way, start at the outside of the row and begin to dig the line. Hopefully your loose garden will allow for easier digging than regular soil. The first plunge of the implement should be deep and then gently pry up the soil. Be careful with a shovel, which can easily cut roots, it is very unforgiving compared to a forked implement. You will begin to see the mighty roots amalgamated with clumps of dirt, some may be forked and others will appear long like a carrot. By hand, separate them from these clumps for safest extraction. Clip the root from the plant stem if it is still attached then place the root into a container. The extra weight of the stem will not increase the value of the root and it should always be carefully removed. **Do not** remove the neck of the root with the scars during this process.

(i) Washing

Within hours after the roots have been collected from the garden they will need to be quickly washed. This however is just a term of art because you are really just rinsing them off. Leave the small feeder roots and the neck attached to the main root. Never scrub your roots, it may seem counterintuitive but this is how it is done. The *washing* of ginseng roots

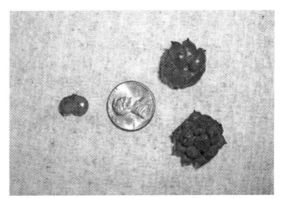

Ginseng Berry (left of Penny) With 2 Goldenseal Berry Clusters (above)

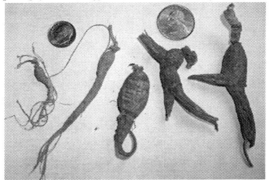

Ginseng Roots, Ages: Seedling(2), 3, 4, 5 & 8-Year Old (above)

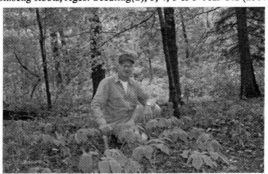

Mature Ginseng Plants Dying-Back in
Preperation for Winter Hibernation (above)

involves running them under gentle running water, merely removing the bulk of soil and debris. The method likely depends on your harvest. Larger harvests can be spread out on screens and carefully hosed down being mindful not to apply too much pressure. Modest harvests can be quickly sunk into dipping troths and placed on screen trays for drying. The method of washing the roots matters little as long as the root skin is not damaged during the process, the root is not to be scrubbed clean, or left soaking in water. You are not selling carrots or another garden vegetable that requires to be cleaned in fact very clean ginseng roots will likely bring a lower price. Expect that soil will be left in the circular rings and wrinkles of your roots this is expected and preferred at auction.

(ii) Drying

From the outset of ginseng trading in North America improper drying techniques marred trade and reduced root values. Not unlike every other aspect of growing this herb there is a balance. Roots dried too quickly by artificial methods can develop a brown discoloration and have a diminished value, those dried too slowly can develop mold and rot.

Again the facilities demanded for this is dependent upon your yield. At least a month if not longer before you dig your fall harvest drying racks should be constructed. Drying trays can be as rudimentary as having the roots placed out on window screens supported by sawhorses or lumber-framed trays with screen attached. The beds of the trays should be made of a material such as screening that will facilitate air circulation and consistent drying of the whole root. The roots should be placed in a single layer, never stack roots on these trays.

Locations for Drying

A drying facility can be simple like an upstairs room in your house, attic, or garage. It must be a place that cannot be compromised by cool (below 70 degrees Fahrenheit) or excessively warm (above 95 degrees Fahrenheit) temperatures. It should also be free of mice, or strange smells such as fuel, which often permeates garages and garden sheds. Smaller roots will be completely dried after a couple of weeks while the larger roots with more girth can easily take 4 – 6 weeks. This is where a room in the house works well for modest growers because keeping an upstairs room at 70 – 95 degrees (Fahrenheit) for up to six weeks in the fall is easier than a shed or garage. Keep several thermometers located in different corners of the facility or room monitoring the temperatures. Small heaters can work well just make sure they are not spiking the temperature levels above 95 degrees and most importantly make certain they are not a fire hazard. Also any direct heat source like the rays of the sun coming in through a window should not be allowed to touch the roots. Generally it is wise to inspect the drying process every day or two to make sure mold or anything else is not attacking them.

Avoiding Moisture

During the drying process your roots will shrink and become limp, as nearly 2/3 of their body weight dissipates. With thousands of roots emitting moisture in an enclosed area a dehumidifier is an excellent addition to the process. However fans may alternatively be added. Good ventilation can be achieved with window fans during the day expelling the moist air especially in warmer climates. Be watchful of rainy and damp fall weather while drying. Wherever you decide to dry your roots, be it a shed, garage, room, or whatever, it must be kept warm and dry since mildew and mold are only too willing to make an appearance.

C) Storing And Selling

From soft and flaccid roots in the beginning, over the course of the drying process they should become hardened and be able to snap when done. Check a few of the roots having generous thickness if they are light, dry, without any pungent smell, and feature a white center when snapped open then it is time to store them for marketing.

(i) Storing

Never employ storage containers that are airtight because this will encourage spoilage, simple and clean reinforced cardboard boxes or cardboard drums work best. The cardboard container top can be sealed because the material breathes. Before removing the roots from the trays and placing them into the containers take pictures for insurance reasons.

After the roots are placed into the cardboard box or drum they must be stored in a dry setting accompanied by a suitable room temperature. A basement is fine as long as it is not damp, also make sure they are stored in an insect and rodent free environment. Amazingly ginseng can store for years in these conditions as long as it was properly dried and all the while maintaining its commercial value. However sitting on thousands of dollars of dried roots for several years is not advisable because fire, theft, and water damage could easily filch those roots from you.

(ii) Selling

Small cultivators and wild diggers can sell to the local fur buyer. You likely will not get the best price but it offers the least effort. However for medium and larger operations it is best to contact an established ginseng buyer. Once you have dried, documented, and inventoried your harvest it is time to consider soliciting the help of an exporter or buyer. These operations can be found on the Internet, you can inquire at the place you purchased your seed or root stock, or sometimes you can call the local county extension of the Department of Agriculture and get help finding a reputable buyer depending on how knowledgeable that branch is. Also for the growers, by this juncture you have been growing ginseng for at least 4 – 5 years, likely longer, take the time to join a ginseng growing society. Usually the meetings and newsletters will offer uniquely provincial information that is exceedingly helpful especially with locating a reputable buyer.

Depending on the buyer and where they are you may have to send your roots through the mail. Communicate and establish what the buyer prefers before sending any roots. Strong cardboard boxes work fine for this. Always insure your roots. Also check with the department of environmental conservation in your state and make sure you are not running afoul of any state and federal regulations if you plan on mailing your ginseng out of state. Always document all transactions and the dates of all conversations or letters of correspondence not only for taxes but in case a dispute arises. It should never happen, but in case it does, be prepared.

Finally do not try to dump poor, damaged, mangled, discolored, or moldy roots on a buyer. Besmirching your reputation as a grower will not prove helpful. Furthermore these buyers inspect tens of thousands of roots every year before exporting them so it would be silly to think that you can fool them. The small percentage of roots that are not fit for the market can be consumed. An excellent treat is to place a root in the refrigerator and cut off a dime-sized slice daily to eat with a meal.

D) Grading

Ginseng prices are far from static. Basic economic principles of supply and demand like with any commodity are at play. If you are selling wild roots you have to compete with a shrinking supply in the wild and the black market sale of wild ginseng, field cultivated sellers are consistently seeing their prices dwindle, while woods-grown and woods-simulated enjoy a buoyant market. But there is more to the ginseng root than the method of how it was grown. The Asian auctions will scrutinize the roots and judge them on a wide range of criteria including the size, color, shape, texture, health, and taste of the root just to name a few. There are almost forty grades, which is far more complex than the simple taxonomy of wild, woods-simulated, woods-grown, or field cultivated. When the time comes to sell discussing the grades with your exporter after they have initially inspected your lot of roots will provide you with more clarity.

Chapter IX

Growing Goldenseal

Goldenseal makes an outstanding complimentary crop with ginseng especially if you are already equipped for ginseng production. The two enjoy compatible growing conditions however goldenseal in most cases is even more resilient and versatile.

A) Goldenseal The Herb

Goldenseal (or *Hydrastis canadensis*) is an herbaceous perennial from the Asteraceae family. It enjoys a similar habitat as ginseng, preferring rich well-drained soil and growing under the hardwood canopy of the forest with 65 – 80 percent shade. The herb gets its golden color from the prevalence of berberine, an antimicrobial. This imbues the roots and fibers with a yellowish gold hue. Its vast geographic range and golden color has inspired other names by which it has been sometimes called such as: orange root, tumeric root, wild circuma, ground raspberry, eye-balm, yellow root, and yellow pucoon. The natural range however has been shrinking due to the wild populations being harvested for profit.

(i) The History
The original majority of the geographic areas for goldenseal did not stretch as far north as ginseng. Its traditional native habitat stretched from Minnesota, Michigan, Vermont, and southern New York, south to Georgia and west to the Mississippi. Similar to ginseng, goldenseal prefers shaded woodland with rich soils but unlike ginseng it can also be found in shaded meadows, hedgerows, and even thickets.

Goldenseal Plant & Root

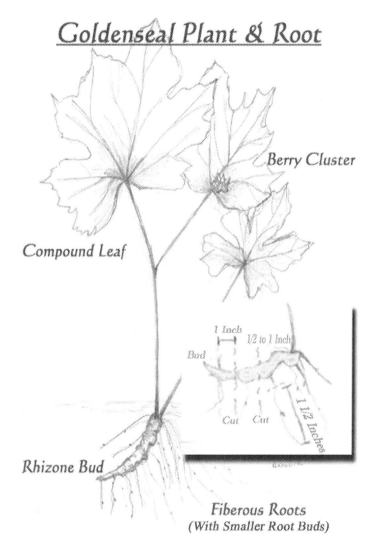

Berry Cluster

Compound Leaf

Rhizone Bud

Fiberous Roots
(With Smaller Root Buds)

The commercial market for goldenseal in North America was greatly developed in the 1860s. However by the 1880s the over-harvesting resulted in a documented reduction of wild plants. Although in the early 1900s domesticated cultivation was begun, wild specimens have continued to be removed and their natural presence is steadily shrinking. Eventually as with ginseng, the federal government acknowledged the dangers of goldenseal exploitation and it is listed in Appendix II of the Convention for International Trade on Endangered Species of Wild Fauna and Flora. This treaty endeavors to regulate and monitor the sales and export of threatened as well as endangered species.

Goldenseal is easier to grow than ginseng, seems virtually impervious to the common diseases that assail ginseng, and generally it can be harvested sooner. The price paid per pound is significantly less than wild, wild-simulated, or woods-grown ginseng, but lately it has been close to the prices offered for field cultivated ginseng and goldenseal requires substantially less work. Goldenseal even transplants very easy, the only major enemy seems to be animals both four legged as well as two legged.

Historically the use of goldenseal was very common among the indigenous natives of what is presently the eastern United States and such use is well documented. The Cherokee Indians used it to make dyes, health tonics, and for the treatment of snakebites, whereas the Iroquois Indians thought it was helpful with treating pneumonia. Both settlers and Iroquois Indians ingested the root to remedy digestive problems. Berberine, canadine, and hydrastine are the alkaloids in goldenseal that are believed to be the medicinal constituents. These properties include most notably the berberine as an anti-bacterial, the canadine as a sedative, and the hydrastine, which helps with circulation as well as smooth muscle contractions.

(ii) Goldenseal Today

Presently as an herb it is one of the most popular selling in America and for good reason since it has a plethora of presumed healing qualities and applications. Today some of the more common medicinal claims are its ability to be an effective treatment for: oral sores, eye problems, hemorrhoids, as well as an anti-inflammatory, diuretic, digestive stimulant, and reputedly aids the body by placating swollen mucous membranes during a respiratory infection. Notwithstanding the pharmacological applications of goldenseal, it does have toxic qualities and should not be consumed raw like ginseng. The side effects of consuming too much raw goldenseal can range from mouth lesions to convulsions caused in large part by the hydrastine. Goldenseal should not be ingested while a woman is pregnant because it is capable of causing a miscarriage. Many experts believe that if it is taken in a pill-form, it should not be used for long periods of time. Nonetheless despite these claims it still remains a valuable cash crop.

B) The Life Cycle

Naturally the propagation of goldenseal occurs through successful germination of its berries and a creeping underground root system that facilitates the spread of new stalks creating a thick patch in several years if the conditions are favorable. The roots offer growth in two ways through rhizomes budding and long thin wormlike fibrous roots budding that extend from the main root (or rhizome). From these buds, plant stems emerge and this dense growth after six years can engender the main root to rot away freeing the connected plants from the parent root at the epicenter. Indeed in nature this would be a waste of a very marketable root but it prevents the goldenseal patch from smothering itself. Artificially propagating goldenseal is realized through harvesting and planting seeds as well as exercising various techniques at cutting and multiplying the root using these buds.

(i) The Berries
The berries of goldenseal look very different than ginseng. Goldenseal berries look almost like a raspberry mixed with a cacti flower from a distance. The seed cluster emerges with a white and green flower in May or June. Eventually the mass turns into a green cluster, then red, and eventually a deep red that

has a very slight purple tint to it. By late July or early August the deep red berries will descend to the ground or be consumed by animals. A mature berry cluster can easily contain 20 small, hard, black seeds within it. Their size will be slightly smaller than a BB or a round unground piece of pepper. The range of 10 – 30 seeds is considered the standard. If the berry falls onto the ground and becomes covered with natural mulch the seeds after winter are capable of germinating that spring or may even go into dormancy and emerge the following spring. Harvested or purchased seed should be planted in the fall before the ground freezes.

(ii) The Plant

Goldenseal is a perennial and the plant tops begin to grow usually by late April or early May. The stems grow from buds on a horizontal rhizome that can be as long as six inches depending on the age. The rhizome will have a girth of ½ - ¾ of an inch in diameter, be covered with a brownish exterior skin, and have a bright yellowish color on the inside. Around the rhizome will likely be an abundance of yellowish smaller fibrous roots, which also may have diminutive buds that lead to new plants.

Seedlings growing from a seed offer initially only a generic leaf, while in the second year a true palmate leaf emerges (similar in appearance to a grape leaf). A plant that is at least three years of age and healthy should have two stems that emerge at the same point on the root raising between 8 – 16 inches in height. The palmate leaves offered are not easy to describe, but look for 1 – 3 compound leaves that are broad, possibly ten inches in diameter, and project out like lobbed fingers, with serrated edges.

By late spring or early summer a solitary flower develops on the plant where the leaf meets the stem. Blooming can last for a couple of days or a couple of weeks contingent on environmental factors. This greenish white flower measures around ½-inches wide and does not have any petals. It does however contain about a dozen pistils and several dozen spreading stamens. Usually by the middle of the summer the pistils give way to a small berry cluster. The green berry cluster will turn red by the end of the summer, slightly resembling a raspberry. A healthy plant can yield as many as thirty seeds and at that point of the growing season the plant top is nearing its end and will soon begin to die back. It is interesting to note that over 90 percent of the upper plant's development is finished in the first month of the growing season of that year.

If left on their own, the rhizomes and smaller fibrous roots will keep horizontally spreading out and new plants will emerge from the buds formed on these roots. Eventually a patch will develop with closely growing plants.

C) Planting

Before planting it would be wise to take a moment and contact the local branch of the Department of Agriculture to make sure that a permit is not first required for goldenseal cultivation. A few states are starting to pursue this and it is always wise to be safe than sorry. Cultivation in the woods should work well in the natural range that goldenseal originally grew in, as well as geographic zones with similar environments to the original locations like the Pacific Northwest.

(i) The Site

If you are using goldenseal as a replacement crop in former woods-grown ginseng beds, then it is likely that you need not worry about selecting another site. Otherwise if you are looking for a specific plot for goldenseal then the plot chosen should be very similar to ginseng. Moist, rich, loamy, soil that offers efficient drainage, such as a location on a slope is preferred. Companion plants for goldenseal indicating favorable growing conditions are preexistent include: ginseng, blood root, mayapple, and black cohosh.

Shade

The easiest shade to procure is under a hardwood canopy, which is ideal. Although a random conifer mixed in should not be a problem, a majority of deciduous trees present is really needed such as: ash, basswood, cherry, hickory, iron wood, oak, poplar, and walnut. As discussed with ginseng, elms are great for shade but the danger of them succumbing to Dutch elm disease and leaving open holes in the shade canopy is too great to allow a grower to depend on them. Artificial shade can be constructed using wooden lath, snow fence, or polypropylene, and lumber but the cost of construction may not be justified by the yield. Nonetheless for more detail on artificial shade construction refer to Chapter II, Section (iv). Whatever shade is utilized it should be around 65 – 80 percent. If more than 80 percent shade is present the development suffers, goldenseal seemingly can stand slightly more light than ginseng.

If you choose to construct artificial shade consider removing it during the winter if you encounter sizable snow accumulation, which might cause it to collapse.

Drainage

Clay soil should be avoided because goldenseal requires adequate drainage. If after working with the soil it feels gummy in your hands, during regular weather, it would not be ideal. Consider adding large amounts of sand, leaf mold, and small stones if you are determined to plant on a given site that is compromised by high amounts of clay

Soil

The soil pH can be as high as 7.0 but the 5.5 – 6.5 range is better. Do not expect goldenseal to endure the vast pH range that wild ginseng can. Fertilizer should be kept to a minimum perhaps just a shot of Miracle-Gro sprayed early in the growing season. Amendments discussed in Chapter III can be considered but goldenseal is not nearly as fickle as ginseng. Having the soil analyzed at the local university or county cooperative extension for your goldenseal crop is an option but if a location is chosen in the woods with existing companion plants it is likely that it will yield good goldenseal crops. The more favorable the soil, the healthier and more prolific the plants will be. Topsoil rich in humus (organic matter like dead leaves) is ideal because it prevents the soil from fusing together as it holds the minimum moisture required while porous enough to allow the excess to drain through, and it is comprised of ideal nutrients.

If you have to add natural material to improve the soil, shredded leaves, rotted saw dust, and compost can be used as long as they are well decomposed. Otherwise they may steal nitrogen from the garden site as they rot also immature compost may call unwanted attention from small animals. Add these materials into the top six inches of the soil while rototilling, as needed.

(ii) Method

Clear woodlands and create gardens just like one would do with woods-grown ginseng and in the same manner as described in Chapter IV. Dig down with a rototiller six inches below the surface and be ready to add rotting forest leaves into the soil if it lacks the desired rich texture. Then plant, cover with soil, and apply mulch.

Mulching

Mulching provides a protective shield against loss of moisture, weed growth, and extreme temperatures. It should be about two inches in depth during the winter and light by the time spring arrives to accommodate the plant. Shortly preceding the emergence of the plants, remove any excess mulch leaving only ½ - 1 inch covering on the gardens, which is a bit less than ginseng. Shredded leaves work far better than straw, which can hold too much moisture and slugs, and better than just sawdust alone. Since goldenseal does not naturally prefer the more northern parts of the United States and southern Canada if you live in these locations consider heavier mulching during the winter, 2 - 3 inches is advisable.

When to Plant

An intriguing aspect of goldenseal is that it can be planted with seeds, root cuttings, and even rhizome splitting. The best time to plant goldenseal is during the generous window in the fall stretching from the middle of September until the first frost. Early spring will also work, ideally late April or early May.

Although not ideal, goldenseal roots and root cuttings can be planted later in the spring and even the summer if the opportune moment is missed. With rootlets, place them in a refrigerated or cool place (do not let them freeze) packed in a plastic Zip-loc style bag with a filler like potting soil to help hold moisture, until you can get them into the ground. This will safely buy you some time (several weeks), but the risk is always present that the vitality of the rootlets to grow when finally planted will suffer.

Seeds

A mature plant will usually yield up to thirty seeds, which should be planted in the fall after a seedbed or garden is prepared. Late September and early October is a good time for this.

De-pulping

Before the seeds are planted, they must be de-pulped if picked from existing plants. De-pulping can be accomplished in many ways by rubbing the berries onto a screen thus shredding the berry and freeing the seeds, or gently mashing them with your hands, or squishing them in a container. The method employed may depend on the amount of berries you need to process. Upon picking out the seeds from the squished berry pulp, place the seeds in a container soaking them in water for several days. This will help the pulp further separate from the seed. Unlike ginseng, if there are some goldenseal seeds floating they are not necessarily bad seeds therefore do not throw them away. However look for discoloration. The healthy seeds should be shiny, black, and hard, not white or tan, conventional wisdom demands that these off-color seeds should be jettisoned (although it never hurts to hastily throw them under ¼ of an inch of soil in a little plot in the woods). After separating the bulk of the pulp from the seeds and soaking, promptly lay them on a newspaper and briefly let the air circulate over them so they are dry to the touch. Do not however let them dry out. Then either store them in moist sand like the ginseng stratification box (*see* Chapter V) or more ideally prepare to plant them.

Goldenseal seeds are capable of germinating the following spring or waiting a year. Rates of seed germination are difficult to extrapolate any knowledge from. The success rate fluctuates from a handful of new plants to well over 50 percent the next spring. For best results, if the seeds can be planted that fall, try gathering the seeds, de-pulping them, soaking for several days, and briefly store them in moist sand. During this short storage, keep the seeds in moist sand at a constant temperature of 67 - 73 degrees (Fahrenheit) for at least four weeks until the fall planting.

The successful germination rate will not equal ginseng so planting dense is recommended. These little seeds transplant very easy if the seedbed becomes too crowded. They can be planted in the spring or fall but the fall is highly recommended. If the seeds are spending the winter in a stratification box, like with ginseng, make sure the box is properly buried in a natural and not excessively wet location.

Planting Seed
(5 – 7 years → Roots Are Suitable To Harvest)
Goldenseal seed must be sown in shallow soil, only ¼ - ½ deep. Plant a seed every 1½ - 2 inches in the rows and keep the rows separated by six inches. Cover the seeds with a ¼ - ½ inch of soil and then if sowing in the fall cover them with a mulching

of two inches preferably of shredded leaves, continuing to avoid the use whole leaves as mulch. This mulch is primarily for protecting the seed during the winter. In late April or early May before the growing season begins the following spring, remove all but a thin ¼-inch layer of mulch. These plants need all the energy they can muster to emerge and thick mulch will surely prove to be too much of a barrier. Once the plants go dormant after the first growing season, it is time to transplant the rootlets to gardens or wait a second year if the seedlings are not too dense. Goldenseal grown from seed may take 3 – 4 years before it produces a flower but it should produce a bigger root after five years than a root grown from a cutting. A plant grown from seed should be a suitable specimen to harvest in 5 – 7 years.

Rhizome Division, Root Cutting, and Rootlets

Whether you are purchasing goldenseal rootlets or expanding the existing stock of your garden, this versatile herb can be grown from dividing its own root in several different ways. Naturally this may extend the timetable of growing a marketable rhizome but the objective here is to expand your growing stock or create rootstock-product to sell.

A mature root of four years of age can usually be cut into three new roots or perhaps as many as five new smaller roots, but the success rate might suffer. With this you must exercise prudence and much depends on what you have to work with as far as the health, available buds, and fibrous roots attached to the existing rhizome.

After only one or two years this new plant, from former rootstock, should be mature enough to yield berries. Unfortunately sometimes these plants grown from dividing an existing root may not expand as quickly as a seed-grown plant. This is because the newly divided plant continues on believing it is the mature parent plant. Refer to the Goldenseal Diagram as needed for clarification on the anatomy of the plant and its rhizome.

Rhizome Division
(3 – 5 Years → Rhizomes Are Suitable For Harvest)

A rhizome is a subterranean root that has smaller bottom roots attached. When your plants have at least two years of age dividing the rhizomes is an excellent way to expand the gardens. The cutting of the rhizome should be done in the fall when the plant goes dormant. With a sharp clean knife and cutting board you will go about separating the root into pieces that offer the best chance of future success. Obviously this must be done in an orderly manner that will not allow the roots to dry out.

After extracting the root from the ground, carefully remove any excess dirt and debris so that the small buds on the rhizome can be observed along with the large yellow bud. First look for the large buds and from their tip measure ¾ - 1 inch down the rhizome that is attached to it and vertically sever that piece at the ¾ - 1-inch mark. Second with the remaining rhizome in hand look for any small buds. Cut the rhizome into ½ - ¾ inch pieces that have small buds growing. It would be best that each root section have some healthy smaller roots attached with the small bud as well. Promptly plant these root pieces in prepared gardens.

These new plants may be ready for harvest in 3 – 5 years. If you have rhizome pieces left over that do not have any buds on them they can be promptly replanted or if the plant is of a suitable size and age (4 – 6 years old) it can be cleaned, dried, and made ready for sale. Yet one more option if this operation is carried out in early spring can be to replant and divide the root after it sprouts new buds, which is covered under the section on *Layering*.

Root Cutting
(4 – 6 Years → Roots Are Suitable For Harvest)

The goldenseal root has smaller fibrous roots attached to the main rhizome. Early during spring these smaller roots that developed yellow buds can be removed in two inch pieces and planted under ¾ of an inch of soil in a special bed for the summer. By the fall the root pieces that have developed plant stalks can be dug and placed into regular gardens.

Rootlets
(4 – 6 Years → Roots Suitable For Harvest)

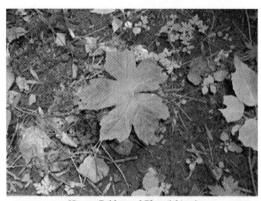

Young Goldenseal Plant (above)

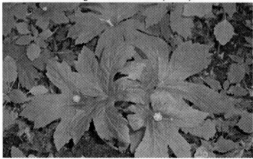

Mature Goldenseal Plant With Developing Berries (above)

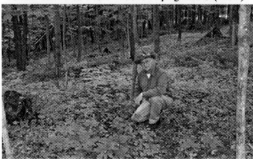

Example of a Healthy Woodsgrown Goldenseal Garden (above)

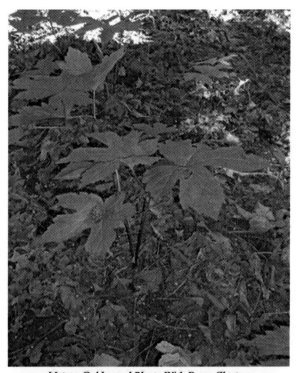

Mature Goldenseal Plants With Berry Clusters

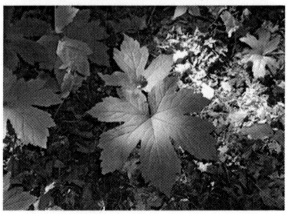

When transplanting rootlets from a seedbed or if purchased from a seller abide by the same depth, spacing, and mulching directions covered under the section, *Planting and Spacing*. Take note that when the rootlet is placed in the row, before covering it with soil try not to let the smaller fibrous roots become congested and massed together.

Layering

This technique requires some skill and may be best if undertaken initially for reasons of fun and curiosity. The term has been used for both rejuvenating the rhizome piece devoid of any buds and working with the smaller fibrous roots covered under *Root Cutting*.

Although a rhizome piece not having a bud should form one eventually and begin to sprout a stalk if simply replanted, it can also be placed in soil and held in a temperature range of 50 – 60 degrees (Fahrenheit) to facilitate faster growth. If the outside temperature will not allow this, then the technique may even be accomplished by constructing a planter out of wood and setting the operation up in your basement.

When a yellow bud is observed growing then the rhizome-piece can be planted like a typical rootlet in a garden otherwise leave the bud-less rhizome in the controlled soil mixture and check it again in a week or two.

Planting and Spacing

Rootlets and root cuttings should be planted in prepared ground every 6 – 8 inches, in rows that are 8 – 10 inches apart. Two plants every square foot creates a good concentration. The depth to bury them depends on the size of the rootlet. The dug row should be deep enough whereby the buds on the rootlets, facing up, are covered with about an inch of soil and covered with a one-inch layer of shredded leaves or straw.

Also simple sulfur powder available at almost any drug store should be applied to the cut sections of rhizomes before they are replanted. This dry powder will help facilitate healing and prevent root rot by sealing the oozing cut on the root. It makes a rudimentary band-aid. Furthermore when dealing with roots, rootlets, and rhizomes, always take care not to allow them to dry-out during the process unless of course the roots are being harvested for sale as dried root

D) Maintaining Healthy Goldenseal

Aside from abiding by the same **SDS (Shade, Drainage, Soil)** formula as covered earlier (*see* Chapter II), goldenseal should develop few of the diseases and troubles encountered with ginseng. It can endure a drought but if the lack of rain is severe the plant may wilt back and go dormant early. Goldenseal does require slightly more rain than ginseng but for small/medium forest-based growers, especially those already successfully cultivating ginseng, worrying about irrigation is overkill. If you are attempting to grow large amounts of goldenseal in a traditionally arid environment, then commercial irrigation equipment like a water pump, tanks, hosing, and piping should be considered.

(i) Disease
Disease creation and spread will always be hastened by close planting and wet/humid conditions. Forest-grown goldenseal will encounter very few outbreaks compared to the petri dish setting of commercial growing. The close cramped humid conditions of artificial shade have yielded reports where some commercial growers are claiming that traditional ginseng maladies are now attacking goldenseal (e.g. Alternaria, Fusarium, and Rhizoctonia). These are developments that all growers will simply have to wait and see and be watchful of. The worst affliction of ginseng, Phytophthora cactorum, does not seem to attack goldenseal despite some anecdotal reports by growers believing it "may" have. Although it could easily have

been misconstrued as Phytophthora when in fact it was Botrytis-based dampening-off.

Root Knot Nematode

An important early step in growing goldenseal for large commercial operations that are creating gardens in former fields might be to have a test conducted on the soil to make sure you are not inundated with root knot nematodes if you have reason to believe they are present or you live in a region where they are a known problem. There seems to be a higher prevalence of them in warmer regions. If unchecked, they will rain devastation upon goldenseal roots.

Botrytis

Traditionally it has been the more common of the overall rare afflictions attacking goldenseal. At first it may be a blister-like lesion on the leaves or stem, then it becomes a grayish and velvety patch. All parts of the goldenseal can be attacked from the berries to the rhizome. If left unchecked the plant can wilt, list over, and die if it is young. The removal of the afflicted foliage of the plant and replacing the surrounding mulch is effective, but once the velvety patch of spores appear the chance of transmission is greatly increased. If it is sanctioned by your local regulations, fungicides that kill Alternaria may prove somewhat effective to spray the area with.

(ii) Other Factors

Compared to ginseng there is much less to be concerned with when cultivating goldenseal especially if the garden is grown under a natural shade canopy. Aside from disease, paying attention to the following should help keep your crop healthy.

Airflow

For woods-growers keep the brush and lower branches of the forest canopy trimmed allowing the best possible ventilation.

For commercial growers, try to keep the framework for the artificial shade at least 6 – 8 feet from the ground. Also have openings in the structure that allow the ingress and egress of the prevailing winds circulating new air in throughout the gardens before naturally exiting.

Slugs, Moles, and Mice
These pests will bother goldenseal in the same manner they damage ginseng. For treatment and eradication refer to Chapter VI Section (vi).

Grower's Tip!
If you are planting goldenseal in a former ginseng bed that was decimated by Phytophthora consider the risks of opening up the fungi-imbued soil for cultivation if other ginseng beds are still in the immediate vicinity.

E) Harvest and Sale

Goldenseal has a harvest routine very similar to ginseng but with less growing time and hardly any spraying the herb almost raises itself.

(i) When to Harvest
Unlike ginseng, which can live for decades and maybe centuries under ideal circumstances (a root exceeding 100 years old was reputedly found in China in the 1980s), goldenseal needs to be harvested or it will stymie itself. The time to harvest is usually 3 – 6 years after the plant began growing. Typically after five years or maximum six, the center root will not grow any larger. As with ginseng, harvesting should be carried out in the fall after the plant begins to enter its natural dormancy unless you are also selling the tops then they must be harvested green shortly before beginning their natural die back.

If the plants are in the lower end of the marketable age (3 – 4 years old), before digging the roots, it is wise to extract some at random from gardens earmarked for harvest ensuring that they are a suitable size. If the roots are satisfactory, then carefully rake off all the remaining leaves, mulch, and debris in the garden. The roots should be carefully dug with a spade or similar implement. Take your time not to damage the smaller fine roots attached to the main rhizomes. Cautiously clean the roots of excess soil and material that is not part of the root (and leave the root fibers attached). Any large buds that are chosen to be removed from the harvested rhizomes should be promptly planted or placed in temporary storage containers where they cannot desiccate. Do not plant them in the same bed that is being cleared.

(ii) Cleaning the Roots

The larger roots that are being sold should be thoroughly cleaned with water but not damaged in the process. Proper washing can be accomplished by placing them on screens and hosing them down with a gentle enough stream so as not to damage the rhizome and fibrous roots. Root washers of a commercial grade can be purchased, or if the soil coating on the root is loose enough they can be dipped in large tubs filled with water for a short duration and then placed on drying racks comprised of lumber frames with screen trays.

(iii) Drying

For this step set the roots in a dry and stench-free location. If a garage, shed, or barn is chosen be aware of ambient smells that should be avoided like gasoline. As the roots dry check them frequently to make sure that they are not being disturbed by rodents, mold, or uneven drying. Always avoid drying temperatures that are too high, too low, and too inconsistent. A constant level of 80 degrees (Fahrenheit) would be good, even 90 degrees may be acceptable but the key is to not force the roots to dry too quickly. If the outside dries and becomes hard it protects the moisture in the middle of the root preventing the rhizome from properly drying. If you are experiencing a spell of weather filled with humidity consider adding fans to circulate the air in the drying room. After a week they should be substantially if not completely dried. When ready for storage the roots should take on a dark brownish-yellow tint and will have lost over 70 percent of their initial weight from when they were dug. A sweet and distinct aroma will accompany this drying process. When the root is believed to be sufficiently dried, check a few as samples, you should be able to snap the rhizome with your hands.

(iv) Storage and Selling

After the roots have completely dried they should be stored in drums or containers made of cardboard or simple but sturdy boxes with the top taped shut. Avoid plastic because it does not breath. A dry room with stable temperatures (cooler is best) that is free from rodents and pervasive undesirable smells such as: fuel, tobacco smoke, or solvents should be appropriated for storage. The dried root can easily be stored for months.

The price paid at auction and by buyers is based on the market fundamentals of supply and demand. Obviously you should never try to peddle wretched roots. Unlike ginseng with its entrenched grading system, goldenseal prices generally are broad and fair. Finding a buyer may be accomplished in many ways such as: inquiring at the local branch of the Department of Agriculture of known buyers, asking sellers of goldenseal seed/ rootlets, checking with your local fur and ginseng dealers, or talking to local farm co-op members, all are great places to start. There are also some buyers listed in the Appendix.

Chapter X

Things to Consider

This field guide is packed with as much information as could reasonably be included to be imparted onto you the reader and perspective grower. While we endeavor to include as much as possible, so much more simply must be learned by experience. The relativity of ginseng growing conditions alone will require constant fiddling to find what works best in your gardens. Some of you will have more trouble than others based purely on the land you have to work with. But as has been covered, much can be overcome by adhering to the **SDS** formula, amending the soil, doming flat ground, and even if need be utilizing artificial shade. There are some other miscellaneous ideas that a new grower should attend to.

A) Becoming Resourceful

Once the basics are put to memory on growing and caring for your crops you may find yourself always thinking of new ideas or ways to make something easier and more economical. One way is to be resourceful. Many plastic containers either thrown away weekly or sent to be recycled can have useful purposes. Especially milk, vinegar, windshield-washer fluid, or most 1-gallon plastic containers mentioned earlier, which are great for storing water (after they are thoroughly cleaned out). Some smaller plastic containers hold seed very well, or make good slug traps with only minor modifications.

Also with a black felt-tipped marker and a measuring stick mark lines on the handles of some of your garden tools every inch, like a shovel handle (especially if already painted white), a measuring device in the field can be very helpful. Other simple but industrious ideas involve using old clothes and lumber to construct scarecrows and pie tins hung from trees to help spook animals as they flutter in the wind. Or another example is saving old window screens to make drying racks, as you can see there are many household items that can be of use.

By far one of the most important things a grower can do is record their actions in a logbook. Computations are needed to be carried out anyway, deciding everything from how much slug poison you will use in a season, to the amount of seed that is warranted to be ordered (or sold), or garden space available that needs to be cleared.

Keeping track of gardens may seem easy at first, but after several years and thousands of feet under cultivation it can all begin to blend together without good notes. Also your data that is extrapolated will be far superior to anything else you can learn from another grower. This field manual is the best guide we can provide to get you started but the real journey begins after your plants break ground and you apply what you have learned and begin to deduce what works best. A logbook is also necessary to keep an accurate inventory of your supplies, which may be seasonal in nature and difficult to replace in the middle of the growing season if you run out. Furthermore if you decide to run the operation as a business keeping good records will be a necessity. Finally do not rely purely on a computer hard-drive for your logbook without the information that is stored being backed-up and also saved on disks. Although it is rudimentary, a standard composition notebook is still an excellent choice.

B) Setting up as a Business

Growing ginseng and goldenseal for profit can be a rewarding project, hobby, or secondary income and thus you should take the time to contact the Secretary of State's office of your respective state and consider filing your business. Each state has different requirements and fees which can be sorted out by either a phone call or checking the homepage of your state on the Internet. The advantage of filing as a business, especially a simple partnership, helps ensure that reasonable expenses incurred are tax deductible. For large operations a Limited Liability Partnership (LLP) or a corporation may offer preferred advantages such as shared but limited risks, spread among various business partners.

C) Economic Opportunities Other than Dried Roots

The preferred paradigm is to harvest and sell the mature roots of your crop attaining the best possible price when the time is right. However there are other options. If for some unforeseen reason the land holding a garden has to be disgorged from your operation or a health crisis forces the scaling back of the growing, planting, and maintaining of the gardens, there are other means to generate income.

(i) Selling Rootlets
The rootlets of both ginseng and goldenseal can be sold. The prices paid for rootlets differ from year to year and from seller to seller but it is an option, obviously the older the rootlet the higher the price paid. First make some calls or conduct some searching on the Internet and locate a reputable commercial operation that would like to buy them. If you have the resources you could try to sell them yourself by taking out an advertisement in an outdoors magazine like *Fur-Fish-Game* or attempting to sell them online with either on auction site or a website but this may get tiresome. The options and prices offered all have to be weighed when making that decision. Rootlets should be dug in the fall when the plant goes dormant and then promptly stored in a cool moist medium until they reach their destination. Make sure they do not dry out.

(ii) Selling Seeds

The prices offered for goldenseal seed are much lower than for ginseng. Although any grower could pursue this option it would make more sense for medium to larger scale ginseng growers to consider it. One healthy acre of mature ginseng (assuming it is at least in its third or fourth growing season) could offer conservatively 100 pounds of viable seed per year. If you stratified and sold the seed at a low price of $60.00 per pound that equals $6,000, or you may want to keep half of your seeds and sell the other half. However remember these are numbers assuming that everything goes well and things do not always take that course. Nonetheless, selling extra stratified seed is a very real option, you could also sell it "green" but your profits would be considerably less. Again your options are selling the seed on your own or selling the lot to a commercial ginseng seller.

(iii) Selling the Plant Tops

When selling the green plant tops to both ginseng and goldenseal make sure you pluck the top at the absolute end of the growing term thus giving the root the maximum chance to grow that season, but the top must also still be green. Marketing the tops may be more difficult than finding a buyer for roots, seeds, or rootlets, but tops are purchased for use in teas, creams, and tonics. With ginseng plant tops, the buyer will not want chemical residue on the leaflets so if you secure a buyer make sure this is planned into your spraying routine. Chemical residue on the leaves is not typically as problematic with goldenseal because often it needs little if any spraying.

D) Final Thoughts

Any agricultural endeavor runs the risk of being imbued with both success and failure. We recommend trying this as a supplemental income at least initially, which allows you to treat this as a hobby.

Occasional disappointment will be incident on the journey from seed to harvest. As long as the risks are understood, anticipated, and preferably avoided, the experience should be a rewarding one. Best of luck and be sure to check the appendix for helpful information as well as updates on our website:

www.GrowingGinseng.org   or

www.GrowingGinseng.org/bookupdates.htm

(for book updates)

Appendix

Vendors

The following list of sellers and buyers of seeds and roots is given to help you get started. We have sifted through dozens of sellers to provide a sample of those with fair prices. It is however paramount to do comparison price shopping. Prices can be almost double from one vendor to the next as demand outpaces supply for regional sellers. Therefore contact **at least** 2 – 3 from this list before you order so you establish a fair market price.

"Best" American Ginseng
PO Box 606, 337 South 3rd Street
Bayport, MN 55003 (USA)
E-Mail: sales@GotGinseng.com
http://www.GotGinseng.com

Buckhorn Ginseng
23855 Buckhorn Lane
Richland Center, WI 53581 (USA)
Phone: (608) 647-2244

Horizon Herbs
PO Box 69
Williams, OR 97544 (USA)
Phone: (541) 846-6704
E-Mail: hhCustServ@HorizonHerbs.com
http://www.HorizonHerbs.com
[Siberian Ginseng, large selection,
organically grown, prices may be higher]

Hsu's Ginseng Enterprise, Inc.
Paul C. Hsu, T6819 Co. Hwy. W.
PO Box 509
Wausau, WI 54402-0509 (USA)
Phone: (715) 675-2325
E-Mail: info@Hsu.ginseng.com
http://www.English.HsuGinseng.com

Mickey Hare
R.R. # 1 Waterford
Ontario, Canada N0E 1Y0
Phone: 519 443-5948
Fax: 519 443-4492
Cellular: (519) 428-8497
http://www.kwic.com/~hareginseng/

Mountain Top Farms
PO Box 231
Owego, NY 13827 (USA)
Phone: (607) 760-2179
E-Mail: sales@mountainfarm.com
http://www.MountainFarms.com

Northern Tool + Equipment
PO Box 1499
Burnsville, MN 55337-0499 (USA)
Phone: (800) 533-5545
Fax: (952) 894-0083
http://www.NorthernTool.com
[seller of equipment not seeds]

Ohio River Ginseng & Fur, Inc.
PO Box 2347
East Liverpool, OH 43920 (USA)
Phone: (330) 385-1832
Fax: (330) 385-1842
E-Mail: info@OhioRiverGinseng.com
http://www.OhioRiverGinseng.com

Premier Ginseng and Herb Company
PO Box 395
Marathon, WI 54448 (USA)
Phone: (877) 825-3627
E-Mail: GinsengSeed@aol.com
http://www.GinsengSeed.com

Roots "O" Gold
Box 92
LeCenter, MN 56057 (USA)
(507) 665-6310

Finally when finding a seller sometimes those that invest the least in advertising offer the best prices. Checking the classified ads in an outdoors magazine like *Fur-Fish-Game* will often avail you to several venders looking to sell ginseng seed or goldenseal rootlets far below the prices found on Internet websites.

Do not forget to check www.GrowingGinseng.org for our updated list of vendors.

Ginseng Garden Spacing

6,500 – 8,500 Seeds in Every Pound

Gardens: 1 Seed Every 4 - 5 Inches in Rows 6 – 10 Inches Apart

Seedbed Spacing: 1 Seed Every 1 – 1½ Inches in Rows 6 – 8 Inches Apart

Transplanting Rootlets: 1 Rootlet Every 6 – 8 Inches in Rows 8 –10 Inches Apart

100 – 300 Mature Roots = 1 Dry Pound

Quick Disease Reference of the Most Common Diseases

Systemics Protect Plant from the Inside, Fungicides Kill Disease on Contact

1 Tablespoon per 1 Gallon = 1 Pound per 100 Gallons

Regular spraying, proper drainage, and good air flow will help prevent all of the following:

CAUSE	SIGNS	TREATMENT
Alternaria	Papery brown lesions **WITH** yellow hallow	Remove plant top Spray Fungicide
Botrytis	Grayish patches on leaves, berries, and stems	Remove diseased part Spray Fungicide
Dampening-Off	Small lesion on yearling's Stem with the plant bent over	None, the plant dies Spray/Replace mulch
MSD	Reddish tinge on the edges of the leaves. Usually in 2-year olds. Root is dark and malformed.	None, the plant dies
Phytopthora	Reddish, yellowish, brownish, blister-like lesions that turn translucent. The plant wilts. The roots are discolored and reek.	Remove top if only in leaves but if in root promptly remove and all plants in 3 –5 feet. If in the root, the plant dies.
Bugs	Small symmetrical holes on leaves not accompanied with red/yellow.	Apply bug killer with Fungicide spraying
Over Spraying	Uniform Copperish or Goldish tint on leaflets	Consider waiting several more days between spraying

Checklist of Needed and Recommended Supplies

Listed in the order of when they will be needed.

Viable land with good **(SDS)**   _____
Rototiller at least 4½ horsepower   _____
Chainsaw   _____
Branch pruners   _____
Hard rake   _____
Hard soil or Warren hoe   _____
Shovel   _____
Spade   _____
Ginseng/Goldenseal seed or rootlets   _____
Fungicide (Manzate)   _____
Empty plastic containers/ Zip-Loc bags   _____
Fertilizer   _____
Mulch   _____
Slug poison   _____
Rubber gloves   _____
Sprayer   _____
Small Funnel   _____
Systemics   _____
Spreader Sticker   _____
Insecticide   _____

Garden Notes

For easier monitoring of your gardens, photocopy this page and insert the information for each respective plot.

GINSENG	TARGET RANGE	CURRENT LEVEL	AMENDMENTS ADDED
PH	5.15 – 6.66	_____	_____
Organic Matter	5.65	_____	_____
Nitrogen	112.0	_____	_____
Phosphorous	95.0	_____	_____
Potash	235.0	_____	_____
Calcium	1150.0	_____	_____
Magnesium	95.0	_____	_____
Sulfur	69.6	_____	_____
Sodium	35.0	_____	_____
Copper	.50	_____	_____
Iron	234.0	_____	_____
Manganese	4.50	_____	_____
Zinc	2.50	_____	_____
Boron	1.25	_____	_____
Aluminum	75.70	_____	_____
Molybdenum	3.20	_____	_____

GARDEN #_____ LOCATION_____

Date Tested _____

Remember to Check: www.GrowingGinseng.org

CPSIA information can be obtained at www.ICGtesting.com
Printed in the USA
BVOW031336231011

274313BV00001B/37/A